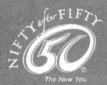

NIFTY *after* FIFTY®

A Guide to Better Aging & Fitness for Men and Women

SECOND EDITION

First edition published as
WIN IN THE SECOND HALF

SHELDON S. ZINBERG, M.D.

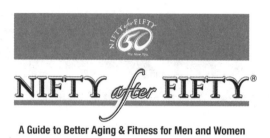

NIFTY *after* FIFTY®

A Guide to Better Aging & Fitness for Men and Women
SECOND EDITION

Production by Laurel Associates, Inc.
Cover by IQ Design
Illustrations by Jim Balkovek

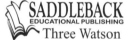

SADDLEBACK
EDUCATIONAL PUBLISHING
Three Watson
Irvine, CA 92618-2767
Website: www.sdlback.com

First edition published in 2003 as *Win In the Second Half*

Copyright © 2008 by Saddleback Educational Publishing

ISBN-10 1-59905-341-1   ISBN-13 978-1-59905-341-7   eBook 978-1-60291-675-3

Printed in the United States of America

13 12 11 10 09 08   9 8 7 6 5 4 3 2 1

DEDICATION

This book is dedicated to all
those who read it and implement
the changes required to be
Nifty after Fifty.

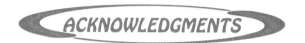

ACKNOWLEDGMENTS

Many people played a role in making this book a reality. In part, it began as a family affair, the initial inspiration coming from my son, Abram. He became genuinely exasperated by my unending and frequently explosive expressions of frustration about the abundant misinformation given to the public on the subjects of aging and fitness. Finally, he said, "Enough is enough, already! If it bothers you so much, write a book that separates the facts from the myths." And so I did.

My wife, Nancy, was an indispensable asset as a research assistant and as an *ex officio* editor. More importantly, the book could not have been completed without her encouragement and her gracious tolerance of my peculiar hours of toil.

My daughter, Perri, has a doctorate in psychology. Her opinions and input on the sections dealing with dementia, mental exercise, and sexual behavior in the mature adult were enormously helpful.

The thousands of health experts, research scientists, and authors who have previously written on these subjects furnished a fount of information from which well-founded opinions could be formulated and articulated.

Last, but most assuredly not least, I wish to thank all of my colleagues, friends, and patients for their invaluable opinions and ideas. Most deeply, I wish to thank my patients. The nature of their problems and how we dealt with them together was the most inspiring impetus for this writing.

CONTENTS

FOREWORD

WELCOME!

Every one of us will get old or die young. To put that thought in better perspective, please note that neither "old" nor "age" is a four-letter word. Recent research has cast a new light on the so-called aging process. Our better understanding of this inevitable experience gives the information in this book enormous importance—both to you as an individual and to society in general.

We're all aware that the effect of aging baby boomers on American demographics will be astounding. By the year 2010, there may be more people between the ages of 54 and 74 in this country than between the ages of 24 and 34, and by the year 2050, there may be more than one million people over 100 years old! All of the evidence suggests an amazing increase in longevity for many, if not most of us. During the next 20 years, the number of people in their 70s and 80s—and even into their 90s—seems likely to increase exponentially. Those of you now in your 40s and 50s will have a much longer life than you probably anticipated—and certainly longer than the life expectancy of previous generations.

In short, more of us will age, and more of us will age even more. That's both the good and the bad news. While the good news gives us many reasons to rejoice, at the same time the bad news gives us some important reasons to be concerned.

We've all seen it happen: As we get older, we encounter chronic disease, decreased mental ability, and a loss of physical strength, along with reduced acuity of our senses: taste, touch, smell, hearing, and eyesight. How many of these potential losses will *you* experience, and how soon will they happen? A great deal of that answer is genetically determined. Genetics, however, is not the *only* determinant of how you will age. In fact, it accounts for 50 percent or less of the process.

Environmental factors—including the air you breathe, the food you eat, the amount of physical and mental exercise you get—will determine 50 percent or more of how you age and how long you live. Genes may load your gun, but your environment pulls the trigger. Much of your own aging process is under your control. After all, *you* choose the food you eat and the amount of exercise you do (or do not do). *Your* choice of lifestyle makes up the greater part of your environment— and good choices can delay or even reverse many of the effects of aging.

If you've already made a series of bad choices, I urge you to believe this: *It's not too late*—it really isn't. No matter what your age is, you can get mentally and physically stronger, become more energetic, more vigorous, more resistant to disease, and have a much happier and healthier life. The information in this book can help you achieve this goal—*but the choice is yours*. Today is the first day of the rest of your life, and you can decide what you want that life to be like. If you want to "win in the second half"—or even in the last five years of your life—this book will show you how to do it.

Where did I get this information? It's a summary of what my patients have taught me in the privacy of the examination room over the last 35 years. One thing I've learned is that people are far more likely to make life-affirming decisions and stick with them when they thoroughly understand the scientific fundamentals underlying their concerns. Simply stated, when you understand something, you are more likely to accept it and to embrace the implications flowing out from it. To that end, *Nifty after Fifty* carefully and clearly explains the scientific basis of the different aspects of aging. In these pages you will learn how aging affects the cellular and molecular nature of your mental and physical makeup. Even more importantly, you will learn how to positively modify these changes through a detailed and thorough discussion of metabolism, diet, nutrition, herbs, supplements, and exercise.

Don't be distressed about growing older! Read on to discover the life-changing improvements that you can still achieve. By following the simple, safe, and thoroughly enjoyable programs I recommend for mental and physical exercise, you'll be surprised to discover how quickly and positively you can address concerns ranging from everything from skin to sex.

Sheldon S. Zinberg, M.D.
January 2008

THE CHALLENGE

Getting old isn't for sissies.
—Bette Davis

Forty is the old age of youth;
fifty is the youth of old age.
—French proverb

Remember when we were young? We could hardly wait for the trappings of mature adults! But we changed our minds as the years went by, didn't we? Like generations before us, we had no idea of what was coming. We couldn't imagine ourselves in less than prime condition, mentally and physically. Then time took its toll and the bad news slowly began to dawn on us in the form of depleted strength, energy, and mental acuity. This progressive loss of physical and mental fitness is the greatest challenge to our continued functionality, our quality of life, and our future independence—our ability to stay out of the nursing home. Most importantly, it's happening to all of us—*right now.*

The good news is that most of these changes can be delayed, many can be prevented, and some can even be reversed—if we start *right now.* It's true. Whether we live to be 50 or 98, staying healthy, independent, and functional is *not* an impossible dream. The goal is to compress morbidity—to die as young as we can but as late as we can. The fact is that by becoming and staying as physically and mentally fit as possible, we can prolong a much richer quality of life and enjoy more lasting independence.

IT'S NOT TOO LATE

Obviously, the best time to have started this process was when we were young, but now is the next best time. Whether we admit it or not, many of us have given up. We're convinced that the damage is done, that it's too late to make a difference. If that's what you think, you're wrong. We've all seen our favorite football or basketball team blow the first half of a game and then stage a dramatic comeback to win the game in the second half. The game of life is no different. No matter how badly we might have played in the first half, we can choose to stage a comeback and be *Nifty after Fifty.*

No matter how slow we've been to get started, we can adopt appropriate behaviors to steadily improve the condition of our minds and bodies to delay, prevent, or even reverse many problems that will otherwise compromise our future. Because knowledge is power, it's important to understand our bodies, how the parts function, and what happens to us over time. Whether you have but one year or 50 or more years left to live on this earth, it is never too late to harness this power to improve the zing, the zest, and the overall quality of your life.

MUSCLE WEAKNESS (SARCOPENIA)

Between 20 to 30 percent of older Americans are classified as "frail" because of mental and/or physical deterioration. Many in their 40s or 50s don't even realize they're well on their way to losing their independence. Some may be experiencing *asthenia*, a general sense of weakness. In others, a decrease in bone mineral density (*osteopenia*) may be starting. Usually this gradual decline is the result of simple inactivity and poor eating habits, often magnified by illness—heart problems, lung problems, arthritis, or a combination of similar ailments.

But there is usually one factor that overshadows the rest. That factor is muscle weakness—the common denominator that most often lands us in a nursing home. Between the ages of 45 and 60 we lose one percent of our muscle strength every year. *Sarcopenia* is the medical term used for this age-related muscle deterioration. This accelerates, between the ages of 65 and 75, to an annual loss of one-and-a-half percent of our muscle strength. Almost all of us are or will be significantly weaker at the age of 70 than we were at 40. That change can be very dramatic. Some of us will lose 50 percent or more of our muscle strength between the ages of 45 and 75! Hard to believe? Well, it's true.

Another way to look at it: By not being able to open that jar of jam or jelly, you might save yourself from some extra calories! On the other hand, quite suddenly, you might not be able to get up from the toilet seat.

WE CAN CHANGE THIS

In a recent study, women placed on a twice-weekly strength training program for one year became biologically younger by 20 years. By the end of the study, they were 75 percent stronger, had increased the bone density in their spine and hip areas, had improved their balance, and were far more active in their daily lives. These women had also gained three pounds of muscle and lost three pounds of fat. (Because a pound of muscle is much smaller in volume than a pound of fat, they had become slimmer and more shapely!)

And here's an amazing fact: *There appears to be no age limit on our ability to improve with resistance training.* Studies of men and women between the ages of 80 and 90 who used resistance training two to three times a week showed exciting results. In just six to ten weeks they improved the strength in their legs by more than 100 percent. Some of them even threw away their canes and walkers. Imagine that! These were people 80 and 90 years old. In less than three months, resistance training, like weightlifting, made a huge difference. None of these people became a Mr. Universe, but these results are indeed encouraging. Perhaps this poem explains it better.

Sarcopenia

Sarcopenia—that's its name.
Sarcopenia! Is the devil to blame?
It's sarcopenia that makes us frail,
And sarcopenia that makes us fail.

With each new page
Of advancing age,
In hardly a blink
Our muscles shrink!
Each muscle spindle
That begins to dwindle
Is the power leak
That makes you weak.

At first it's asthenia,
Then osteopenia.
But it's just the beginning:
When our bones start thinning,
We shuffle and trip
And break a hip
Then use crutches to roam
Through some nursing home.

But we can beat this
And we will defeat this
With the strength we gain
In the muscles we train.
Their fibers will coil
With exercise toil
And our strength will grow
From the effort we sow.

Then all will witness
Our replenished fitness
With zest that flowers
From our newfound powers.
We then can revel,
"Be gone, you devil!
We're now much greater—
And we'll see you later!"

So, you see, it's not too late—not by a long shot. You can prevent the plaques in your arteries from getting bigger. In fact, you can make them smaller or perhaps even lose them entirely! You can make your arms and legs and your bones stronger. You can improve your energy level, your memory, your balance, your stamina, and your flexibility.

In regard to our brains, physical exercise has been shown to improve cerebral circulation, brain growth factor, and mental acuity. When combined with specific mental exercises, your thinking skills and your ability to remember can be even further enhanced. In short, you can feel better, look better, and actually *be* better. The best news of all is that you can accomplish all this very quickly.

SELF-ESTEEM: OUR ABILITY TO CONTRIBUTE

How we feel about ourselves—our sense of self-worth or self-esteem—is crucial. This feeling is usually rooted in our continued ability to make a contribution—whether it's to our family or friends, our community, or our business. Our "purpose in life" is often what makes us feel most alive, appreciated, and productive. Surely, the successful progress of our lives cannot be measured by how many miles we can walk or whether we can do push-ups. But at the same time it's obvious that the stronger our physical and mental abilities remain, the longer we will be able to go on making contributions—and feeling good about ourselves.

LOOKING BACK, LOOKING FORWARD

CHAPTER 1 REVIEW • • •

- It's true that our physical and mental abilities decline as we age.

- It's also true that we can delay, prevent, and even reverse most of these changes through our own efforts to achieve and maintain fitness.

- In spite of starting late, we can all be "Nifty after Fifty" through a program of regular exercise.

- Muscle strength can be dramatically improved in a short period of time; mental acuity and self-esteem increase along with muscle strength.

CHAPTER 2 PREVIEW • • •

- Is the quality of our aging determined more by our genetic code or our lifestyle?

- What happens to the human body as it ages? Are scientists making any progress in halting or treating age-related disabilities?

- How can we alter our environment to remain strong and independent for as long as possible?

ABOUT AGING

You are never too old to set another goal or to dream a new dream.
—C. S. Lewis

To me, old age is always 15 years older than I am.
—Bernard Baruch, on his 85th birthday

INCREASING LONGEVITY

There are hundreds of theories on aging. Many have scientific merit, but all need more study. One thing is clear, however: *We human beings are living longer.* Some 100 years ago, the average lifespan was 45 years; since then, it has increased by more than 50 percent! Scientists have good reason to predict an even greater increase in the next century.

Sound farfetched? Perhaps the old tongue-in-cheek remark, "If I knew I was going to live this long, I would have taken better care of myself," was less a joke than a fair warning. Why? It's conceivable that the average human lifespan at the end of the next century will be 100 to 120 years—and that those fortunate centenarians will maintain the functional status we now observe in the average 75-year-old!

THE BEGINNING OF AGING

The notion that we start to age from the minute we're born is commonplace but inaccurate. *The fact is that aging is simply the biological balance of the accelerating and decelerating rates of growth and repair.* It might surprise you to know that, in humans, this rate starts to change between the ages of 11 and 25. This marks the beginning of aging—the point at which the accelerated rate of tissue growth and repair begins to slow down. So you see, my friends, the old saying that "life begins at 40" just isn't true. In many instances, however, life really does begin to *show* at 40!

GENETICS AND ENVIRONMENT

The genome (genetic code) of different animals and plants is an important determinant of longevity. The differences in living things are amazing. Some turtles, for example, can live for centuries. Some varieties of rockfish live 150 years, and a few hardy trees can go on living for 5,000 years!

The longevity determinants in genetic codes are extremely complex, however. Consider this comparison: Some 98 percent of the genes in humans and chimpanzees are the same. So why is it that humans live twice as long as chimps? Comparing people to other people is also instructive. Although 99 percent or more of the genetic code may be identical from person to person, the variation of one percent or less is more than enough to make our journeys through life highly individual.

What a big difference one percent can make! We all know individuals who have a family history of longer lifespans. So we're not surprised when descendants of those families also have long lives. On the other hand, we know folks who have a family history of early death due to genetically transmitted diseases such as heart disease, neurological disorders, certain types of cancer, and diabetes. (Diabetes, as an example, may accelerate the aging process by as much as 30 percent.) Genetics can also be a determinant of the strength of one's immune system. A good example is what happened during the bubonic plague epidemic. Millions of people died, of course—but others who were equally exposed either survived the disease or never contracted it at all.

There's no question that your individual longevity is influenced by your genetic makeup. But it also depends on the environment to which you are exposed. As an example, think of two different kinds of flowers—one that thrives in sunlight and one that thrives in the shade. If we place them both in the sun, the shade-lover may wither and die as it shrinks from excessive sunlight. Conversely, if both were placed in the shade, the sun-lover would fail to thrive.

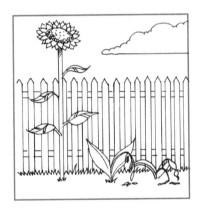 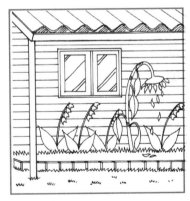

The importance of environment is hard to overstate. In humans, these environmental factors are multiple. They include such things as the nutritional value of our diet, the inhalation of toxic fumes or tobacco smoke, our exposure to free radicals, and a sedentary rather than an active lifestyle. These and many other environmental factors act on our genetic "inheritance" and seem likely to be more than 50 percent responsible for determining our longevity and the morbidity (suffering) that we will or will not experience—just as the sun or shade helped or hurt the different kinds of flowers.

It is the combination of our genetic makeup, our environment, and our lifestyle that determines our longevity. The positive changes we can make in our environment and lifestyle will add life to our years as well as years to our lives. In other words:

> *The human genome*
> *May shape your dome,*
> *But you're the crafter*
> *Of what comes after.*

OUR CELLULAR MAKEUP: DNA, CHROMOSOMES, AND GENES

Every one of us is made up of millions and millions of cells that repeatedly divide to replace themselves. This process of cell death and replacement continues throughout life at such a rapid rate that we are almost completely made anew every one to seven years—talk about makeovers!

At the center of each cell is its nucleus, which contains our DNA (deoxyribonucleic acid). Within our DNA lie the chromosomes that contain thousands of genes—our entire genetic code. The DNA in the nucleus of our cells manufactures the RNA (ribonucleic acid) that makes up the cytoplasm, the part of the cell outside the nucleus. As age advances, however, every time a cell dies it is *not* always replaced by a new cell. If that

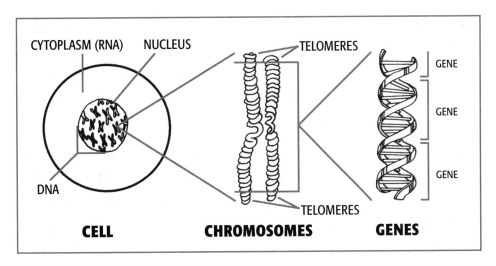

were so, we would never change. We would look the same on the outside; we would be the same on the inside; we would never get older; and we would live forever—but this is not the case. When cells no longer divide to replace themselves, we lose cells—and we age. And as we age and more and more cells die that are not replaced, we finally die.

Cells have their own biologic time clocks that determine how many times they can divide to replace themselves. This biologic time clock consists of tiny substances at the ends of each of our chromosomes. They're called *telomeres*. The longer the telomeres, the more times the cells can divide to replace themselves—and, therefore the greater the potential for a long life.

HOW TELOMERES WORK

With each cell division, the telomeres decrease in length. Shorter telomeres are associated with a decrease in the potential number of cell divisions and potentially, with a shorter life.

Longer telomeres are associated with an increase in the potential number of cell divisions and potentially, with a longer life. Now here is some *very, very* exciting news: A recent study comparing the exercise habits of identical twin brothers and sisters showed an important association between exercise and the length of their telomeres. In this study, the molecular youth of cells appeared prolonged by 4–9 years, depending on the frequency and intensity of the exercise—the more exercise, the longer the telomeres. As many of us have suspected, exercise may be tapping in to that sought after fountain of youth.

It appears that a substance called *telomerase* regulates the length of the telomeres. The more telomerase the longer the telomeres can maintain their length, and therefore, the more times the cells can divide to replace themselves. Our ability to inhibit telomerase, may at some time in the future, offer a cure for cancer. Why? Because cancer cells seem to have an overabundance of telomerase. If it were found that specific types of telomerase would affect specific telomeres, we could conceivably have the best of both worlds. We might be able to stimulate and prolong the life of some cells *and* inhibit the life of cancer cells. The scientific community isn't there yet but anything is possible. It's an exciting prospect.

REALISTIC MEDICAL POTENTIAL

Now that scientists have completed the map of the human genome, there may well be a dramatic acceleration of wonderful discoveries that will have a positive effect on longevity and morbidity. Consider the following: Altering the genetic code of certain worms known as *nematodes* has doubled their lifespan. And, when the genetic code of the fruit fly was altered, its resistance to heat and cold was improved, its physical performance was enhanced by 500 percent, its ability to mate increased tenfold—and its lifespan also doubled!

In recent years, scientists have found ways to rearrange DNA. This involves some very complicated techniques that splice chromosomes and infuse them into bacteria with the use of viruses. These techniques produce what is called *recombinant DNA*, which can be used to alter the genetic code of a plant, an animal, or a human. Our knowledge of this process has already been used to diagnose certain genetic diseases, to replace defective or disease-causing genes, to add protective genes, and to produce special pharmaceuticals such as human insulin. Some diseases are already being treated this way, and I suspect that many more will be treated this way in the future.

PROTEINS AS MESSENGERS

It has recently been established that special proteins act as messengers that may activate or govern the activity of genes. Learning more about what these specialized proteins do may enable scientists to develop drugs to control genetic activities. Some agents that actually decrease blood vessel growth have already been discovered. By depriving cancer cells of blood, this discovery may have an enormous effect on treating that terrible disease. Others agents that increase blood vessel growth have also been discovered. Some of these may be highly useful in treating heart disease and other circulatory problems.

STEM CELLS—HYPE OR HOPE?

Developments in stem cell research have great potential to improve the quality as well as the length of life. Indeed, they may revolutionize the way medicine is practiced! A stem cell, like the other cells in our body, has a nucleus. It contains all of our DNA. But unlike our other cells that have already differentiated into specialized cells—such as skin cells, muscle cells, bone cells, and the like—stem cells have not yet completely specialized into these different types. While all of us have stem cells, the most abundant sources are found in the early stages of the developing embryo and in the placenta. These less mature stem cells seem to have greater potential to specialize into a wider variety of cell-types than more mature or adult stem cells.

Researchers have recently developed techniques to culture these stem cells outside of the body. Just imagine the possibilities! What if scientists could produce skin stem cells to treat burn victims or nerve stem cells to treat patients with spinal cord injuries or Alzheimer's disease? A host of other diseases might also be treated this way. Much research must still be done before these happy prospects could become reality—but the potential is very exciting.

SUCCESSFUL AGING: THE BOTTOM LINE

When George Bernard Shaw was asked in his later years if he had any advice for young people, he said, "Don't try to live forever. You can't do it." Resist it as we might, decline in our physical reserve and some of our mental function is the inevitable result of aging. *But it's also true that we can significantly modify this process—and get results quite promptly.* Successful aging requires our conscious and continuing effort to prevent deterioration by becoming physically and mentally fit, and to stay engaged with people and with life in general. It's how we deal with our environment—our chosen lifestyle—that acts upon our genetic makeup to determine the quality of our physical and mental future.

CHANGING YOUR ENVIRONMENT

ENVIRONMENTAL STRESS

The opossum provides a telling example of the powerful influence of environment. Why? Because its natural lifespan is precariously short. But when opossums were experimentally taken to an island where there was less predatory stress, their lifespan almost doubled as compared to fellow opossums that were subjected to the predatory stress of their previous habitat (but not eaten). So, here we have an animal experiment that strongly suggests that stress has an important effect not only on the quality of life but also on the length of life.

CALORIC RESTRICTION

It's also been shown that caloric restriction can increase longevity. In one experiment, simply restricting calories increased the lifespan of mice by 30 percent. These slimmed-down mice even performed better than their overfed counterparts. They moved faster, suffered less fatigue, and became more capable of negotiating a maze. The caloric restriction used on these mice, by the way, would equate to approximately 1,700 calories per day for an average-sized person. While reducing our intake of calories may well prove beneficial to human performance and longevity, the precise amount of caloric restriction is not yet clear.

FREE RADICALS AND ANTIOXIDANTS

What other factors cause cell damage and rapid aging? Free oxygen radicals are thought by many to be the major culprit. They are a result of the normal metabolism of oxygen in our bodies—but they're also found as pollutants in the air and caused by excessive sun exposure. Some believe that cigarette smoking and diets high in animal fat can further increase the accumulation of free radicals.

One interesting analogy suggests that free radicals cause oxidative cell damage in much the same way that free radicals in the atmosphere cause iron to rust. In other words, they are believed to cause the cells of our bodies to "rust," to age, and to die. The accumulation of these free radicals has been associated with a wide range of disorders ranging from cancer and cardiovascular diseases to skin wrinkles.

Antioxidants including vitamin A, beta-carotene, vitamin E, vitamin C, and selenium are thought to scavenge these free radicals and prevent their accumulation in the body. Luckily, these antioxidants are abundantly present in foods such as dark green leafy vegetables, carrots, fish, milk, eggs, and asparagus.

The value of antioxidant supplements is still controversial—but since these antioxidants are readily available in such tasty and nutritious foods, why *not* include them in our diet?

LOOKING BACK, LOOKING FORWARD

CHAPTER 2 REVIEW . . .

♦ The trend is clear: In the past 100 years, human life expectancy has increased by 50 percent; even further extension seems inevitable.

♦ The length and ongoing quality of our lives are equally determined by our genes and our environment.

♦ Exciting new research suggests that some beneficial as well as harmful genetic activities may soon come under scientific control.

♦ The conditions of our environment—such as stress and diet—are largely under our *own* control.

CHAPTER 3 PREVIEW . . .

♦ How does the brain work, and what changes occur as we age?

♦ What is "brain growth factor," and how can it be increased?

♦ Is there any way to forestall or counteract memory loss and poor concentration?

♦ Is some sort of dementia almost a foregone conclusion? Why or why not?

3

OUR MENTAL MUSCLE

The brain is the organ of longevity.
—George Alban Sacher

When I meet a man whose name I can't remember,
I give myself two minutes; then, if it is a hopeless case,
I always say, "And how is the old complaint?"
—Benjamin Disraeli

There's no doubt that advancing age causes physical changes in the human brain. But as yet scientists have only a limited understanding of exactly what happens and what can be done about it. There are many mysteries yet to be solved!

OUR NERVOUS SYSTEM: HOW IT WORKS

During the early stages of embryonic development, our stem cells receive a signal that determines their differentiation and specialization. Some cells become heart cells, others become brain or bone cells, and so on.

The specialized cells that make up the brain and the rest of the nervous system are called *neurons*. Neurons have long branches called *dendrites* which make a connection, called a *synapse,* with other neurons. With the help of chemical substances called *neurotransmitters*, messages are transmitted to other neurons and muscles across these synapses. How efficiently these messages pass from one neuron to another determines how well

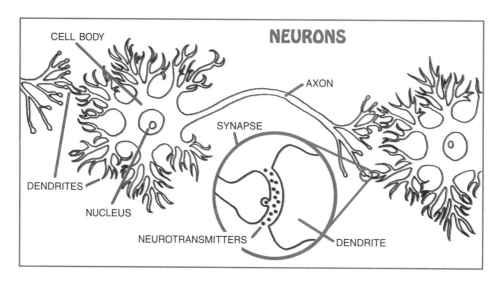

NEURONS

CELL BODY

AXON

SYNAPSE

DENDRITES

NUCLEUS

NEUROTRANSMITTERS

DENDRITE

we think, how we move, and how we recall or remember things. The system works like an electrical circuit. *The important thing is to realize that both mental and physical exercise can improve circulation to the brain, the branching and connecting of neurons, and the activity of neurotransmitters.*

GLIAL CELLS

There are billions of neuron cells as well as billions of other kinds of cells—such as glial cells—in the nervous system. Until fairly recently, glial cells were regarded as little more than structural supporting cells in the brain. The latest research, however, suggests that glial cells may play a crucial role in increasing the growth of dendrites and the number of synapses. Why is this good news? Because this information may have a significant impact on our understanding of brain disease and the treatment of these disorders as we forge into the future.

OUR AGING MINDS

Studies have shown that about half of our mental ability is genetically determined—and not surprisingly, this genetic influence persists into old age. This is true for skills such as memory, problem solving, reading and writing, and the speed at which we think. The other half of our mental "horsepower" is actually determined by our lifestyle—including such factors as diet, exercise habits, and mental initiative.

With progressive aging, there may be a decrease in the number of neurons and dendrites—and thus in the number of synapses or connections. This gradual loss can result in a decrease in abilities such as spatial orientation, deductive reasoning, and short-term memory—that's the bad news. But there's good news, too. *The bad news can be delayed, compensated for, and even, in part, reversed!*

JUDGMENT

And here's some even better news. There are some things the brain does *better* as it ages. As an example, we can make more informed judgments based on our life experience. Some people call this wisdom—using the knowledge we've gained from experience to solve problems. After all, every success and failure we've ever had is an experience. Most of us have learned a great deal from these experiences. When we are able to apply what we've learned, we're ahead of the game.

Sometimes, of course, we can't recall an experience because it's buried too deeply in that magnificent computer called our brain. But even "buried," lessons we learned from experience produce a gut feeling or automatic reflex—often called *intuition*—that serves us every bit as well as if we could recall it. Younger people often discount these gut feelings. Why? Because they're appropriately taught to justify their decisions with logical analysis (and also, because they don't have as much life experience). We can get quite frustrated by what appears to us to be analysis-paralysis—and the reluctance of younger people to accept our judgment. But we need to keep our dismay in check. After all, it was precisely this type of analysis that programmed our *own* mental computers during our youthful days.

It's likely that some of the experience we've accumulated over the years may have little value today. Why? Because of the advent of new technology. But our life experiences with interpersonal relations and how people react to one another don't change over time. Studies designed to test the ability to solve difficult interpersonal life problems showed that older people scored higher than younger people.

The bottom line: *Although we may remember less, we may well understand more.* Even if we do experience more difficulty remembering specific details, we may well have a better understanding of broad concepts.

FORGETFULNESS

A person's memory can begin to decline at the tender age of 16! In most people, however, the ability to remember reaches its peak between the ages of 15 and 25. Memory recall is likely to remain fairly stable into the mid-thirties and then decline at a rate of one percent a year between the ages of 40 and 70. Clearly, this can translate into a significant loss of memory-related skills.

The good news is that lifestyle changes can do a lot to preserve and even improve brain function. A healthful diet, physical exercise, and stimulating mental exercise can improve memory by a factor of 10 to 20 years. In other words, a 75-year-old can regain the ability to remember as well as he or she did at 65 or even 55!

BRAIN GROWTH FACTOR AND EXERCISE

There's no question that we can help ourselves improve our own mental function. How? A chemical substance in the brain called *brain growth factor* can be increased. Both physical and mental exercise appear to escalate neuronal dendrite formation and cerebral circulation as well.

At one time scientists believed that after the brain was fully developed, it gradually and irreversibly atrophied over a long period of years. The assumption was that this deterioration could not be halted or reversed. Now we know that this concept is incorrect. It's a proven fact that both physical and mental exercise can increase brain growth factor, actual brain size, and mental ability.

Recent discoveries indicate that every time your muscles contract they produce a substance called IGF-1. This protein enters the bloodstream, travels to the brain and stimulates the production of brain derived neurotrophic factor (BDNF). BDNF increases the growth of dendrites, neurons, and synapses in an area of your brain concerned with memory (hippocampus) and possibly in the frontal lobes, the area concerned with decision-making, as well. The studies also showed significantly improved memory and problem-solving abilities in the subjects who indulged in regular exercise and increased the production of these wondrous chemicals. Some scientists now believe that regular exercise may not only slow the aging process in the brain—but may actually reverse it.

Here's an example of how mental exercise works: In a large metropolitan area, scientists measured the brain size of recently hired taxi drivers. Two years later, after the drivers learned the street routes associated with their new job, their brains were measured again. A significant increase in brain size was found! The mental challenge of learning new material had actualiy increased their brain size. So let's get with it: Keep thinking and keep exercising. If you're not already doing it, then let's get started.

Mental challenges such as memory games, crossword puzzles, reading, and problem-solving of almost all kinds are examples of mental exercise that can expand the branching and connections of brain cells. Varying our mental activities and taking on new tasks can be particularly helpful. Activities such as volunteering on an advisory committee, participating in discussion groups, taking classes in art or literature—or almost anything that might be of interest to a given individual—can enhance the production of brain growth factor.

Many of us note that with advancing age we don't think as fast as we used to. We don't process new information as well. We forget what jokes or stories we've already told, and find that we're repeating ourselves. As we forget where we left our glasses or the keys to the car or forget a word or a name, we may fear that dementia is looming on our doorstep. But no matter what else you forget, remember this: *You've been forgetting things all your life.*

WHAT'S IMPORTANT AND WHAT'S NOT

The kind of forgetfulness that normally comes with aging isn't necessarily the beginning of something more serious. Too often we get frightened because we know that dementia can be gradual in onset. So the first signs of weakness make us depressed—and then we gradually begin to lose confidence in our capacities. Left unchecked, this loss of self-esteem can catalyze an even further depreciation of self-confidence.

Jumping to unwarranted conclusions is, was, and always will be a big mistake. If you forget where you put your keys, it's not terribly important; we all do that. If you forget to whom they belong, it could be important. If you forget where you put your hat and your glasses, it's not terribly important. But if you put them in the freezer, it could be important. All of us forget the names of some of the people we meet; that's not serious. But if we forget the names of our children or grandchildren, that could be serious. A story I like to tell in this regard goes as follows:

For 20 years a 95-year-old woman and her 90-year-old kid sister had been eating lunch nearly every day on the same park bench. One day the younger woman said to her sister, "My dear sister, there's something that has been bothering me for the last two weeks, but I've been too ashamed to mention it."

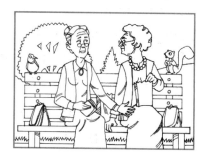

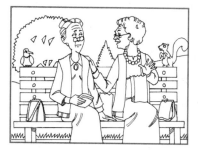

"You shouldn't be ashamed to tell your older sister anything! Tell me what's bothering you. Maybe I can help," the older woman replied.

"Well, for the last two weeks or so I've been trying and trying—but I can't remember your name," the younger woman admitted. "Please remind me."

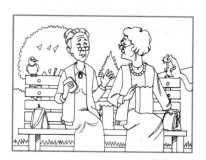

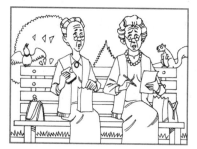

"Surely," said the older sister as she took a pencil and a piece of paper from her purse. She poised to write and then paused. "How soon do you need it?" she asked.

Unlike the sisters in this joke, many of us needlessly harbor and nurture inappropriate fears. In some instances, we can become thoroughly obsessed by these irrational fears—even though the odds are greatly in our favor. The famous words of FDR, "The only thing we have to fear is fear itself," can be appropriately applied here.

Just think about it. Many of our mental lapses are due to simple impatience—which can cause a lapse of focus or concentration. In other cases, it may be that we have become more easily distracted. That only indicates that we need more privacy to assimilate certain types of information. In still other cases, we may have taken stored information so much for granted, we simply forgot it. Let me repeat: *The most important thing to remember is that we've been forgetting things since we were born. Despite advancing age, it's entirely possible for our mental ability and creativity to go unimpaired.*

CREATIVITY

It's true that important innovations in mathematics are most often developed by people in their third and fourth decades of life. By the same token, many innovations in physics and engineering are developed by people in their fourth and fifth decades of life. People in later stages of life, however, have made significant discoveries in the field of biology and produced numerous important works in history, art, and literature. Here are some actual examples:

- **Michelangelo** designed and worked on the magnificent dome of Saint Peter's Basilica from age 72 until his death at age 88.

- **Sigmund Freud** published some of his most important theories between the ages of 65 and 70.

- **Georgia O'Keeffe** painted some of her best works in her late sixties and early seventies.

- **Grandma Moses** (Anna Mary Robertson), a farmer's wife for most of her life, began her painting career in her late seventies.

- **Frank Lloyd Wright** was 91 years old when he designed the Guggenheim Museum.

- **Stradivari** made his best violins in his early nineties.

- **Galileo** wrote his most important scientific theories at the age of 74.

- **Marie Curie** won a Nobel prize for isolating radium in her mid-forties and almost certainly would have continued to make contributions in later life were it not for her untimely death from leukemia.

- **Sarah Bernhardt** continued her brilliant acting career into her late seventies despite having a leg amputated in her mid- to late sixties.

- **Picasso** painted masterpieces at the age of 80.

- **Alfred Hitchcock** directed the movies *The Birds* and *Frenzy* in his sixties and seventies.

◆**Dr. Seuss** was in his eighties when he wrote *You're Only Old Once*.

FIND YOUR INSPIRATION

In my opinion there is a genius buried within each and every one of us, just waiting to be awakened. Because inspiration is the father of creativity, *we must open our minds to recognize and accept inspiration.* The examples I've given just scratch the surface of what the history of creativity can teach us.

Most of us probably don't think of ourselves as especially creative. But we already use creativity in solving problems and making decisions throughout the day. As an example, we adjust our old ways of doing things so we can continue to accomplish certain tasks. This is the thought process of creativity. Perhaps it takes the form of a better way for a teacher to present a subject to the class, or making a more appropriate choice of necktie to wear with a certain suit.

COMPLACENCY IS THE ENEMY OF CREATIVITY

It's a fact that people lose their creativity when they stop caring about things. We greatly diminish our own power when we lose interest or convince ourselves that we can't influence the course of events. What a disservice we do to ourselves when we adopt the complacent attitude of "what will be, will be"! Each and every one of us *can* make a difference. Whatever we do or don't do can affect the outcome of important events. Clearly, the magnitude of the effect we have on many events might be miniscule, but no one can honestly make that judgment in advance of trying. We must avoid "complazyness" and energize ourselves to think and be creative!

THE VALUE OF LEARNING NEW SKILLS

Developing new skills is a great defense against slippage. Activities such as becoming computer literate, surfing the Web, and using e-mail to communicate with friends and family members are mentally stimulating and can be thoroughly enjoyable. The idea that "you can't teach an old dog new tricks" is just as erroneous as "you can't teach a young dog old tricks."

As you age, one of the *most* important things you can do is to learn new skills. The capabilities of a champion bridge player or chess master can be maintained well into their later years. While maintaining such a skill is excellent mental exercise, it is even better exercise to *learn* a new skill.

DISTRACTION AND CONCENTRATION

Many young people can study calculus while listening to hard rock music. Being more easily distracted, we older folk need more solitude to maintain our focus. This is particularly true when we're trying to learn complex material. So take care to avoid distraction when you're attempting to learn new material or develop a new skill. It is the power of concentration that appears to wane with age. And just as muscle power weakens with age and disuse—but strengthens with physical exercise— we can also strengthen our power of concentration with practice.

We must work at it, however. Most people who exercise regularly don't really like to exercise. What they like is the way it makes them feel. Most people who concentrate and study hard don't particularly enjoy it while they're doing it—but they love the sense of accomplishment, the feeling of self-satisfaction, and the way the power of knowledge makes them feel.

Let's be honest about it: As we age, we get lazy in terms of physical exercise and lazy in terms of concentration. But just as we must motivate ourselves to do physical exercise, we must also will ourselves to concentrate; we must *make* ourselves concentrate.

The following story provides an amusing example:

Two brothers, ages 90 and 95, were riding in a car. The younger brother was driving.

"You just passed through a red light. You'd better watch out," the older brother warned.

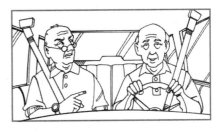

The younger brother, however, drove right on without acknowledging his older brother's concern.

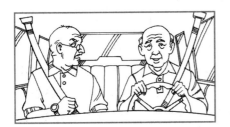

A short while later the older brother again exclaimed, "You passed through another red light! We're going to get a ticket if you're not careful."

But the younger brother kept on driving—again without a reply. Then he passed through yet a *third* red light.

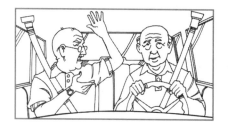

"Are you *crazy?*" the older brother screamed. "Do you want to get us killed? You drove right through three red lights in a row."

At that, the younger brother looked surprised indeed. "Oh, I'm sorry," he replied. "I thought *you* were driving."

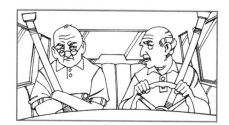

THE CONSTITUENTS OF MEMORY

In order to remember something, you must *learn* that something first. Next you must *store* the information, and finally, you must be able to *recall* it. *Learning, storing,* and *recalling* are the three main constituents or phases of memory. The three processes work hand-in-hand.

THE FOUR RULES OF REMEMBERING

The more thoroughly you learn and understand something, the better you are able to store that information. The more often you repeat something you've learned, the better you are able to reinforce the storage. Likewise, the more often you recall the information, the easier it becomes to recall again—because the storage of that information is strengthened. As an example: Most people can remember the phone number of a friend or a loved one. The more frequently they dial the number, the easier it is to remember. The less frequently the number is dialed, the harder it becomes to recall.

Remembering things is made easier by following four important rules: *repetition, perseverance, patience,* and *BELIEF in yourself!*

No matter how often you fail, you must patiently repeat, persevere, and believe in yourself—because *you can do it!*

DEMENTIA AND ALZHEIMER'S DISEASE

Vascular or multi-infarct dementia is a form of intellectual decline caused by the death of brain cells. This results from the deprivation of blood flow to the brain. Sometimes this form of dementia is caused by multiple tiny strokes the victim hasn't even noticed. This situation is often confused with Alzheimer's disease because both conditions are common in similar age groups.

Most of us know someone with multi-infarct dementia or with Alzheimer's disease. That's why, when we forget something, we may automatically panic that we are entering one of these terrifying dimensions. *Usually, these fears are greatly exaggerated.*

It's true that in some studies of more advanced age groups— as in those between the ages of 85 and 100—the incidence of dementia was found to be as high as 50 percent. But even here, it is important to appreciate that dementia is not an all or nothing process. Some people experience significantly less impairment than others.

WHAT CAUSES ALZHEIMER'S?

If we have a family member with this disorder, we may assume that it is our destiny to be similarly afflicted. While it's true that genetics play a role in early-onset Alzheimer's disease, it's also clear that genes play a much smaller role in later years. Environmental factors such as diet and nutrition, infections, and exposure to toxic fumes have been incriminated. Factors yet to be identified or discovered may also play a significant role in effecting the presence or absence of this disorder—as well as the severity of the disease. *Here again, your lifestyle can be the all-important determining factor.*

Autopsy studies on the brains of people who have had Alzheimer's disease reveal an abnormal accumulation of a type of protein plaques called *amyloid* plaques. As the disease progresses, tangles also develop in the brain cells. It is believed that the accumulation of these plaques and tangles is responsible for the disease, although the precise role they play is not completely understood. Strangely, these plaques have been found in the autopsies of some people who had no symptoms or signs of Alzheimer's disease while they were alive.

Some studies have suggested that the ingestion of aluminum might be a factor—such as the aluminum in some of the antacids we might take for indigestion, or the aluminum in cooking ware.

The jury is still out, however. Exactly how or why these plaques develop and accumulate still puzzles the scientific community.

MAKING THE DIAGNOSIS

The discovery of these plaques at autopsy is still considered the gold standard for diagnosis. Most authorities believe that, in more than 90 percent of cases, the diagnosis in the living can be accurately established by psychological and neurological testing. These tests seek to identify the particular cognitive impairments and structural changes that appear to be reliable predictors of early Alzheimer's.

Recently, the use of a chemical marker combined with a PET (positron emission tomography) scan have been used to identify early changes. This method seems to be highly accurate in diagnosing and predicting the likelihood of developing Alzheimer's disease.

An enormous amount of research continues to be conducted on this disease, and breakthroughs often seem just moments away. Let me tell you of some examples:

- A protein has been found in the blood of Alzheimer's patients that may prove to be an important diagnostic tool.

- A vaccine that showed excellent results in animals is soon to be tested on humans.

- Some fascinating genetic studies appear to have identified five genes on chromosome number 10 that are relevant to Alzheimer's disease. There's good reason to believe that gene therapy may be developed that will cure or prevent the disorder.

Of more immediate interest . . .

- A number of currently used pharmacological agents seem to show promise in delaying the progress of Alzheimer's disease.

- Scientists have also recognized that there appears to be an inflammatory component that occurs in the brains of patients with Alzheimer's. Some researchers theorize that anti-inflammatory drugs, such as those used to treat arthritis, can be of value in delaying the progress or onset of the disease.

In short, there is real hope for those who become afflicted, and it is predictable that this disease, like so many other dreadful diseases before it, will be conquered.

In this regard, there's a little poem about Alzheimer's that I'd like to share with you. It's called "Plaques and Tangles."

Plaques and tangles,
  Tangles and plaques,
Your mind it mangles
  And some it cracks

On chromosome ten
  We found real hope.
We'll search yet again
  While all of us cope.

A vaccine or drug
  We'll soon discover,
From the genes we de-bug
  Or under their cover.

We'll decipher a cure
  From the code of creation,
So try to endure
  While we seek God's salvation.

LOOKING BACK, LOOKING FORWARD

CHAPTER 3 REVIEW ・・・

- ◆ Our "mental horsepower" is determined by both genetics and lifestyle.

- ◆ Age-related memory problems can be improved by changes in our lifestyle.

- ◆ The human nervous system—which controls how well we think, move, and remember—is made up of specialized cells called *neurons* which transmit messages to other neurons via connections or *synapses*.

- ◆ Promising research on Alzheimer's disease offers real hope for future breakthroughs.

CHAPTER 4 PREVIEW ・・・

- ◆ What kinds of learning exercises can forestall a decline in and rehabilitate our mental abilities?

- ◆ How can developing new habits facilitate and sharpen memory skills?

- ◆ What steps can we take to avoid frustration and panic when we forget something?

- ◆ How has neuroscience entered the field of "high-tech brain fitness"?

BOOSTING YOUR BRAIN POWER

*People don't seem to realize that it takes
time and effort and preparation to think.*

—Bertrand Russell

Habits are at first cobwebs, then cables.

—Spanish proverb

The possibilities are truly fantastic! The age-related memory loss (about one percent each year) that usually starts in our mid-thirties can be halted and often reversed. How? By means of physical and mental exercise, we can improve our ability to remember and to think as well as we did 10 or even 20 years ago. These mental exercises (I call them brain aerobics) integrate the three aspects of memory—*learning, storage,* and *recall.* By that I mean we must *learn* something before we can *store* that something. Then, in order to use the information when we need it, we must be able to *recall* what we learned.

Now, nobody's memory is perfect—regardless of age. If those of us who had a photographic memory when we were younger now find ourselves a little short of film—so what? After all, we've been forgetting things all our lives! Our memory of events that happened years ago is often better than our ability to remember who we had lunch with yesterday. In part, this decrease in short-term memory may well be due to a lack of concentration. Or it may be that we are more easily distracted as we age. That only indicates the need for more solitude or privacy to concentrate effectively. Allow yourself the luxury of a quiet place that is free of distractions. This is particularly important when you're trying to learn something new or complex.

Also, bear in mind there are four important rules for learning: *repetition, perseverance, patience,* and *belief in yourself.* Don't lose patience with yourself; repetition requires both patience and perseverance. You can do it! Believe it! Don't sabatoge your own learning process by surrendering on any of these four important principles. *You're in charge.*

USE YOUR SENSES

Many of us learn best by listening to a lecture or a recording. Others learn better by reading or studying with the use of visual aids, such as pictures, diagrams, or videos. Activities such as writing out the targeted material and then saying the words out loud can reinforce our ability to store information and to recall it. If you speak the material aloud, you are, in effect, concentrating on the information and *also* hearing it at the same time. Reading the information, writing it, and speaking it aloud over and over again further entrenches the information in your storage bin, thus improving your ability to recall it. Try to recall the material five minutes later, 20 minutes later, one or two hours later, and then one or two days after that. It really works! The repetition ingrains the material in your storage bin and facilitates its recall. If your goal is to recall this information in the long term, repeat this process in a week or two.

As we go on now, let's use our senses to separate this discussion into different kinds of remembering: learning new material, memory exercises (simple and slightly higher tech), and practical ways to remember things that affect everyday, real-life situations.

LEARNING NEW MATERIAL

Some material can be difficult to assimilate simply because of its complexity. In that case, it can be helpful to write an outline *first*. Then learn the headings of the outline by writing them, reading them, and speaking them aloud. After learning the headings, focus on the material in the first section before going on to the material in the second section, using the same techniques. Be sure to demonstrate to yourself that you know both sections before proceeding to the third and fourth sections, and so on. When you've completed all of the sections of the outline, "take it from the top," as they say in show biz. *Write it, read it, say it,* and *hear it.* Repetition-repetition-repetition.

This technique can be particularly useful with very detailed material such as a contract or an insurance policy, or directions on how to operate an appliance, a cell phone, or a new digital camera. During the learning process it's a good idea to write key questions as you go along. When you're confident that you've learned the material, you can use these questions to test yourself.

Such exercises really *can* improve your learning ability and your memory. Some of you may be skeptical, but believe me, they actually work. How? Practicing the learning and memory exercises in this chapter improves brain function by increasing the branching and the connecting of brain cells, improving circulation to the brain, and promoting the production of brain growth factor. In short, these exercises may result in an astonishing improvement in mental ability. Again—memory skills can be regained to equal what they were 10 to 20 years ago!

MEMORY EXERCISES

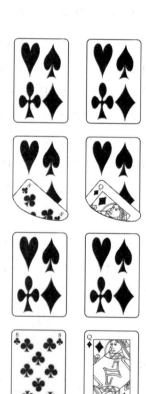

The first exercise makes use of an ordinary deck of playing cards. Place two cards face down on a table. Look at the faces of the cards, place them face down again—and see if you can remember them. Next, repeat this exercise with four cards, placing two on top and two below. Try to remember the four cards before turning them up to see if you're correct. When you have mastered the ability to remember four cards, try two rows of three cards each. Once you have conquered remembering two rows of three cards each, try three rows of three cards each, and so on.

ASSOCIATION

Sometimes the use of an association technique helps us to remember sequences. For example: Let's say that the three cards on the top row are the king of clubs, the ten of hearts, and the queen of diamonds. Making up a simple story can help you to recall the sequence of these cards. Your story, for example, might go like this:

The king of the club gave ten valentines to his queen, who was dressed in diamonds.

Some sequences lend themselves to developing an association more easily than others. When attempting to develop an association proves to be difficult, we may be better served by trying to learn the sequence with raw perseverance and repetition. But I urge you to give association a try. Many people find that merely *attempting* to develop this kind of association can be fun—and it might even improve your ability to be innovative!

POEMS AND JINGLES

Memorizing short poems or jingles is another good exercise. One line at a time can be committed to memory using the reading-writing-speaking technique—or better yet, *reciting*. I suggest you start with short poems (no longer than six to eight lines). If you're successful, try longer poems. (Dozens of books of poems are available in almost any bookstore or on the Internet.) This is not only an enjoyable and effective exercise;

it's also very educational. Imagine the fun of seeing the amazed look on your friends' faces when they hear you reciting poetry—particularly if it's appropriate for a specific event such as a birthday or a graduation. Poems that have a strong tempo and rhyme pattern are especially good choices. Why? Because the tempo and the rhyming will assist you in remembering them.

Short musical jingles that rhyme are not very popular ads anymore—but they are still excellent exercises. They have tempo, they rhyme, and they usually have a catchy tune that aids your ability to recall. Some oldies that come to mind are the old Pepsi Cola and Oscar Mayer Wiener jingles.

> *Pepsi Cola hits the spot.*
> *Twelve full ounces, that's a lot.*
> *Twice as much for a nickel, too—*
> *Pepsi Cola is the drink for you!*

> *I wish I was an Oscar Mayer wiener;*
> *That is what I really want to be.*
> *Cause if I were an Oscar Mayer wiener,*
> *Everyone would be in love with me.*

Some catchy little pop tunes like *Mares Eat Oats* can work the same way. They're enjoyable exercises that have the additional benefit of strengthening the voice and improving your ability to articulate. (Scores of song lyrics are readily available on the Internet.) This kind of exercise recalls something familiar but imprecisely remembered. By refreshing your recall, you will be exercising the pathways that facilitate memory. An added bonus:

Some recent studies suggest that singing may actually contribute to the improvement and maintenance of neural pathways.

Mares eat oats and does eat oats
And little lambs eat ivy.
A kid'll eat ivy, too,
Wouldn't you?

Mares eat oats and does eat oats
And little lambs eat ivy.
A kid'll eat ivy, too,
Wouldn't you?

If the words sound queer
And funny to your ear
A little bit jumbled and jivey—
Sing mares eat oats and does eat oats
And little lambs eat ivy.

Mares eat oats and does eat oats
And little lambs eat ivy.
A kid'll eat ivy, too,
Wouldn't you?

READING AN ARTICLE

Another simple memory exercise is to read and try to retain the contents of a short newspaper article. Once again, this might be better achieved by reading, writing, and reciting it. In this type of exercise, it isn't important to memorize the article, but to practice focusing your attention. After you think you've digested the contents, try to recall it five or ten minutes later. Then try again one or two hours later and once more the next day.

Follow the same process with the poems and the jingles. Try to recall them a week or two later. This technique can further secure the information in your storage bank and strengthen your recall pathways—the routes your mind takes to call up information from your storage bin.

HIGH-TECH BRAIN TRAINING

Neuroscience has entered the field of high-tech brain fitness in a big way! Companies such as Mind Fit, Posit Science, Scientific Brain Training, Happy Neuron, and Nintendo* have developed specialized computer programs that specifically exercise our mental skills. Members of the Nifty after Fifty Center have shown significant improvement by using some of these programs—and they say they're fun to do. The graduated levels of increasing difficulty have been shown to progressively improve memory, speed of recall, and problem-solving skills as well.

---

*For more information, go to: Mind Fit: www.cognifit.com
Posit Science: www.positscience.com
Scientific Brain Training: www.rmlearning.com
Happy Neuron: www.happy-neuron.com
Nintendo: www.brainage.com

REVIVING YOUR DRIVING

It's a fact: As we age, some of our driving reflexes and skills become stale. That's a serious dilemma—because no single factor challenges our independence as much as losing our ability to drive an automobile.

Reviving Your Driving, a program offered at Nifty after Fifty, is designed to resurrect driving reflexes and safe driving habits—and even more importantly, to imbed them in your brain. The program uses computerized driving simulators such as those made by Simulator Systems International or Raydon (The Virtual Driver™). These simulator training courses reproduce almost every kind of weather and traffic hazard imaginable and you can practice them over and over again in a safe environment. When combined with special exercises to improve your reaction time, your ability to focus, stay alert, and concentrate is improved.

People who have used this effective program have become better drivers—and have indicated that it's an enormous amount of fun to use. Almost all of them report measurable improvement in reaction time, problem-solving skills, and attentiveness.

I believe this kind of training can benefit drivers of any age, particularly older drivers and new drivers. It's a very important brain exercise in addition to having an important practical result—*it can save your life and the lives of others*. Try it—you'll like it.

GAMES, GAMES, AND MORE GAMES!

Integrating daily brain fitness training into your life is the best way to stay sharp. Games are an enjoyable and effective way to do just that. Following are a few suggestions:

- Puzzles: Crossword puzzles, word searches, mazes, Sudoku, etc., are great brain workouts. It's a good idea to keep a puzzle book or magazine handy. Don't flip by the puzzles in the newspapers.

- Handheld electronic games: How often do we find ourselves waiting in line these days? Don't let that time go to waste! Pull a game out of your pocket to pass the time and work your mind.

- Game CDs: A single CD can literally provide a lifetime of fun while giving your brain a good workout. Purchase a good puzzle CD that includes a variety of games designed to enhance memory and critical-thinking skills. For instance, the Hoyle Puzzle Games CD includes *Memory Tiles, Mahjongg Tiles, Crossword, anagrams, Hangman, mazes, Star Collector,* various *solitaire* games, and many more. And you can adjust the difficulty level to meet your current needs.

- Online games: The Internet is an amazing source of free memory and critical-thinking games. A search for "free online memory games" could keep you occupied for hours—and mind-sharp for years to come! And don't pass up the games for kids. Some of my favorites are:

  jigsaw puzzles (www.jigzone.com)
  hidden picture searches (www.highlightskids.com)
  Simon (www.lilgames.com/simon.shtml).

THE HABITS OF REMEMBERING

Many very bright young people with excellent brain function not only can't remember where they put their keys or glasses— but habitually forget where they put important documents. (Remember—we've been forgetting things all our lives.) Fortunately, we can develop some useful habits that will help us avoid such common memory lapses. These habits include the use of *organization, consistency, concentration, mental imagery,* and *association.*

ORGANIZATION AND CONSISTENCY

By organizing some of your everyday activities in a logical and consistent manner, you make it much easier to stay on top of things. Example: If you put your car keys in the same pocket each and every time, you are less likely to forget where they are. If you place your wallet or your glasses or any object in the same place each and every time, you will be less likely to misplace it. When you are inconsistent about putting objects in the same places each time, you create the maddening mental task of having to remember where you put them. Give yourself a break. *Develop the habit of consistency.*

Consistency will work even better if you make a logical association between the object and its location. For example, put an insurance or financial document with your other insurance and financial documents. File it away *as soon as you are through reviewing it.* If you want to review it later, you'll know exactly where to find it.

WORK HABITS

Do you sometimes forget to bring your briefcase or some other important item to work? It might be helpful to leave such things in your car before retiring for the evening. Another technique is to leave them in a place where you would fall over them on your way out the door.

It's also smart to make your life at work easier. Don't allow your desk to get badly cluttered. That makes it too easy to get confused and misplace something. Handle the items on your desk one at a time and determine their disposition as best you can at that time.

FENDING OFF FRUSTRATION

If you do misplace something, don't panic. Getting angry with yourself wastes energy. In fact, studies have demonstrated that anger and frustration can decrease your IQ by as much as 30 points! So anger actually makes it *more* difficult for you to remember and function effectively. Try to calmly rethink what you were doing when you last saw the object. Could you have covered it up with a magazine or piece of paper? Frustration and/or panic are distractions you don't need when you're trying to remember something.

MENTAL IMAGERY AND ASSOCIATION

Use some mental imagery every time you put something away. Try to visualize the place you put the item as you're walking away from it. Then, in five or ten minutes, imagine yourself approaching the place where you put the item, and "see" yourself retrieving it. This technique is particularly effective for people who forget where they parked their car. If you leave your car in a large parking lot, *before walking away* take special care to note any landmarks surrounding the vehicle. For example: a lamppost, the entrance to a specific store, the parking level and/or the number of the parking place. Then, as you're walking away from your car, glance back at it and review these relationships. Visualize approaching your car when you're ready to go home. Do this again five minutes later—and again ten minutes after that while you're shopping or taking care of business.

REMEMBERING TASKS AND CHORES

Association and mental imagery are also effective ways to remember tasks on your "to-do" list. If you have to go to the dry cleaners, the grocery store, and the car wash, you might create a mental image of the dry cleaning attendant washing your car and the grocery cashier drying your car.

Always write a list before going to the grocery store! You might also visualize yourself walking down the aisles of the grocery store and looking into your pantry and your refrigerator.

Disciplined application of these simple concepts will soon become helpful habits. The net result? Reducing some of our daily hassles and making life easier.

REMEMBERING NAMES

Many of us have trouble remembering people's names. Why? More than anything else, it's a kind of a benign absent-mindedness that results from a lack of concentration. Although it needn't be, forgetting names is embarrassing for many of us. One technique that I've found valuable is to *repeat the person's name as you're being introduced*. While you're looking at the person, repeat his or her name and try to identify any defining features you might associate with that name. In the course of conversation, repeat his or her name as often as possible. As you walk away, create a mental image of that person's face and associate it with his or her name. Repeat the name to yourself a few times. While not foolproof, these techniques will help imprint the name in your storage bin.

Sometimes nothing seems to help—especially when you're introduced to more than one or two people at the same time. This situation is clearly illustrated in the amusing story of President Clinton's tour of old age homes.

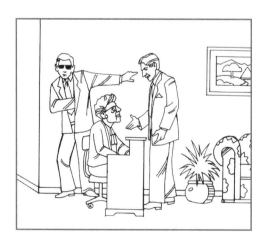

Entering the establishment with his entourage of special agents and news reporters, the president approached the elderly receptionist behind the desk. Facing her eye to eye, he asked, "Pardon me, ma'am. You know who I am, don't you?"

"No, sir, I'm afraid I don't," the receptionist responded kindly. "But if you go down the hall and take a left, somebody there will be able to tell you who you are."

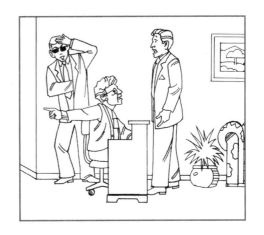

• • •

Think about it. You have everything to gain and nothing to lose. By using some or a variety of these computer and non-computer techniques and exercises, you really can boost the branching of your brain cells, increase the synapses between your brain cells, and generally improve the overall function of your brain! You will be more knowledgeable, more confident, less forgetful, and more empowered. *And you'll love it.*

LOOKING BACK, LOOKING FORWARD

CHAPTER 4 REVIEW . . .

- Memory, learning skills, and creativity often begin to decline as we age.

- By applying the four "rules for learning" in simple mental exercises we can significantly strengthen our weakened skills.

- Memory lapses diminish as we develop new habits of *organization, consistency, concentration, mental imagery,* and *association*.

- Enjoyable high-tech computer programs can sharpen our mental skills and even prolong our ability to drive safely.

CHAPTER 5 PREVIEW . . .

- How does age affect metabolism? Must I resign myself to "counting calories" from here on out?

- Why is exercise so important in a program of healthy weight loss? What's the true relationship between nutrition and exercise?

- Is it a fact that "you are what you eat"? What role do our genes play in determining body weight? How about the influence of glandular conditions?

- Why is it a good idea for us to determine our body mass index (BMI)? Is achieving our ideal weight less important than decreasing our percentage of body fat?

THE TRUTH ABOUT NUTRITION:
Burn, Build, or Blubber

Thou shouldst eat to live, not live to eat.

—Cicero

*The only reason I would take up jogging
is to hear heavy breathing again.*

—Erma Bombeck

THE CONSTITUENTS OF GOOD NUTRITION

It's no secret that excessive body weight can be a very serious health hazard. Why? It increases our risk of developing diabetes, hypertension, heart disease, certain kinds of cancer, and a host of other maladies. At the other end of the spectrum, many of us are malnourished. *All* of us, however, have one thing in common. For those who need to lose weight and for those who need to gain weight—as well as for those who simply want to maintain their weight and be healthier in the process—there really is a magic bullet: a genuine understanding of nutrition and metabolism.

The most important factors that constitute good nutrition have to do with the *calories*, the *nutrient value,* the *fiber content* of our food—and also the use (or abuse) of *dietary supplements.* After considering our different tastes and needs, the next step is to learn to individualize our goals.

CALORIES

Let's begin with the first constituent—calories. Scientifically speaking, a calorie is a unit of energy that raises the temperature of one gram of water by one degree Celsius. Calories are the units of energy in the food we eat—the proteins, carbohydrates, and fats. Our bodily activities can be thought of as the flames that burn these calories. Proteins and carbohydrates have the same number of calories in each gram of weight (four calories of energy per gram). Fats, on the other hand, have more than *twice* the amount of calories in each gram of weight (nine calories per gram). So it takes more than twice the amount of activity—the expenditure of energy—to burn off the calories in a gram of fat than it does to burn the calories in a gram of carbohydrate or protein.

Look at the illustration of a pound of human fat and a pound of human muscle. Be aware that a pound of fat takes up more space in your body than a pound of protein. And it actually has more than twice as many calories as either a pound of protein or a pound of carbohydrate.

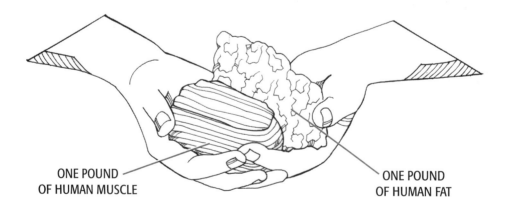

ONE POUND
OF HUMAN MUSCLE

ONE POUND
OF HUMAN FAT

FAT DEPOTS

Including some fat in your diet is important. Certain fats, the so-called essential fatty acids*, are extremely important to good nutrition. And fat produces a sense of satiety or satisfaction. The important thing to remember is that the calories taken in that aren't burned by activity can become body fat. It makes little difference whether the calories come from fat, carbohydrates, or proteins! If you don't burn 'em—particularly carbohydrates— they will turn into body fat, stored in banks of energy called *fat depots*.

Unfortunately, it can be as hard to get the energy out of that bank as getting a loan from First National without collateral! In order to make a "withdrawal" from your bank of body fat, you *must* burn more calories than you eat. When you do that, the calories burned in excess of the calories eaten can be withdrawn from the BOF—the bank of fat.

This fat is distributed throughout the body, but the major fat depots are in the abdomen and under the skin. In the abdomen, the fat is stored between the loops of intestines, and also behind the intestines. Excess accumulation of fat in these areas produces the classical potbelly with which we are all so familiar. Excessive accumulation of fat under the skin produces generous love handles, overhanging rolls of fat on our thighs, a sagging rear end and chest, a redundant neck, and flabby arms.

---

* Examples of essential fatty acids: omega-3 family (fish, flaxseed, and green leafy vegetables); omega-6 family (vegetables, fruits, nuts, and seeds)

CALORIES IN = CALORIES OUT

Some overweight people say. . .

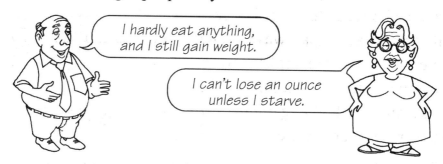

I hardly eat anything, and I still gain weight.

I can't lose an ounce unless I starve.

I don't care what anybody tries to tell you, nobody can gain five pounds by eating a two-pound box of chocolate! The irrefutable fact about both weight gain and weight loss comes down to simple arithmetic: Calories In = Calories Out. With a few exceptions, your weight will always be the result of how many calories you eat and how many calories you burn.

Carefully counting calories and counting grams of food is a full-time job. It's a good exercise in arithmetic—but for most people it doesn't work in the long term. Counting each and every calorie you eat makes about as much sense as trying to count each and every calorie you burn. Practically speaking, neither can be done with accuracy. Our interest should be focused on good nutrition and good weight management. That may mean weight loss for some of us, weight gain for others, or simply weight maintenance for still others. For those of us who should reduce, it must be acknowledged that some people can lose weight more easily than others. This isn't just a matter of will power. It also has to do with individual differences in metabolism.

BURN, BUILD, OR BLUBBER

Proteins, carbohydrates, and fats are metabolized through different but interrelated pathways. The proteins we eat are broken down and absorbed as *amino acids*. These are the building blocks of tissue protein, or muscle.

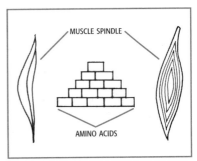

AMINO ACIDS ARE THE BUILDING BLOCKS OF TISSUE PROTEIN—OR MUSCLE.

The fat that we eat is absorbed as glycerol, fatty acids, and triglycerides—or just plain fat. The carbohydrates we eat are

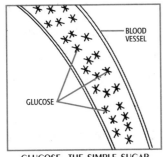

GLUCOSE, THE SIMPLE SUGAR THAT CIRCULATES IN OUR BLOOD

converted to simple sugars. They, in turn, are converted to glucose, the simple sugar that circulates in our blood. This takes place through the digestive process in our intestines and through the metabolic pathway for carbohydrates. Glucose is our source of immediate energy.

Glucose that is *not* used for immediate energy is stored for later use in our liver and in our muscles in the form of a starch called *glycogen*. But what happens if the glycogen in our muscles and liver is *not* used for energy? It, too, can be converted to fat and find a comfy resting-place in our fat depots.

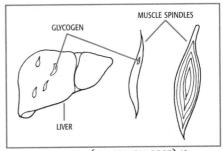

GLYCOGEN (UNUSED GLUCOSE) IS STORED IN THE LIVER AND MUSCLES.

Remember that the glucose in the blood that is not quickly burned for energy must find a storage place in muscle or liver glycogen. If these storage capacities are filled, glucose can also be converted to fat (and join its cousins in a comfy fat depot). So excess carbohydrate calories not used for energy are converted to fat. Likewise, excess protein calories not used for energy and tissue and muscle building are converted to fat. You might call these the interrelated mechanisms of *Burn, Build, or Blubber.*

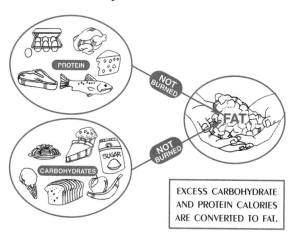

EXCESS CARBOHYDRATE AND PROTEIN CALORIES ARE CONVERTED TO FAT.

DIGESTIVE AND METABOLIC PATHWAYS

In different individuals, some metabolic pathways may be more firmly established than they are in others. So some bodies convert a greater percentage of calories to fat while others convert a greater percentage of calories to building muscle. The varying efficiency of these metabolic pathways may be partly determined by repeated use of these pathways. They may also be partly determined by our genetic makeup, however.

Individuals who eat a large number of calories each day (particularly in the form of carbohydrates) store these calories as fat if they don't burn them through activity. In this way, the metabolic pathway for converting calories to fat becomes increasingly efficient as the metabolic pathways for burning energy and building muscle become less efficient. Conversely, people who increase their metabolic rate by regularly exercising may develop more efficient pathways to burn calories and build muscle.

It's conceivable that the same is true for the mechanisms of intestinal absorption. People who become acclimated to a high-fiber diet tolerate it satisfactorily and are not troubled by excess gaseousness. It's also conceivable that people who eat a high-fat diet develop a more effective digestive process for fats which allows fats to be more easily absorbed and stored in their fat depots. Still, when the rubber hits the road, the bottom line doesn't change: It's Calories In = Calories Out.

THE INSULIN EFFECT

As ingested carbohydrates convert to blood glucose, this rise in your blood sugar level stimulates your pancreas to produce insulin to process the glucose. This is called the *glycemic* effect of food. As an effect of the insulin, the glucose is then either burned as energy or converted to glycogen or fat.

As you might have guessed, carbohydrates such as sugars and starches have the strongest insulin or glycemic effect. The chronic overeating of carbohydrates, particularly sugars, can cause a chronic rise in your insulin level—resulting in the production of more and more fat. Many people who have been overweight for several years are victims of this vicious cycle of events. Perhaps this occurs because of a genetic proclivity. *But surely, carbohydrate overindulgence is a major culprit.* In these individuals, restricting the intake of carbohydrates (particularly simple carbohydrates*) is obviously very important. But it is also important to re-establish the efficiency of the metabolic pathways used to build muscle and utilize energy.

---

* Examples of *simple carbohydrates* are table sugar, fruit juice, white rice, mashed potatoes, all goods made with white flour, and sodas. Examples of *complex carbohydrates* are brown and wild rice, whole-grain pasta, sweet potatoes, beans, green vegetables, and whole-grain breads and cereals.

THE GENETIC EFFECT

We all know overweight people whose whole family is obese. In some cases, this may be due to poor eating and exercise habits that are passed on from one generation to the next. However, we have much more to learn about the role played by genes and hormones in the distribution of body fat and the development of obesity. Research may one day identify a genetic determinant of the efficiency of different metabolic pathways and absorptive abilities of the intestinal tract for carbohydrates, fats, and proteins. Perhaps a genetic proclivity to especially enjoy the taste of certain fattening foods might someday be proved to be important.

A better understanding of some of these issues has been further enhanced by the recent discovery of the *ob* gene and the newly discovered actions of certain hormones. The *ob* gene governs the production of a hormone called *leptin*. This hormone appears to be produced by our fat cells, and its activity serves to *reduce* body fat. On the flip side, the stomach produces a different hormone called *ghrelin*. This hormone *increases* appetite and food intake. It also *decreases* the metabolic rate and the breakdown of body fat. An increase or decrease in the production or activity of these hormones might, at least in part, be genetically determined. Conceivably, all of these and other factors that are yet to be unveiled could interact to make weight control considerably more difficult for some than for others.

An example that makes the same point may be seen in the case of two bodybuilders who eat the same diet and work out equally as hard. One may develop an excellent and very healthy body and the other may become a Mr. Universe. Why the difference? By reason of his genetic makeup, Mr. Universe may have more efficient metabolic pathways for burning energy and building muscle. Again—while it's important to be aware of all of these possible variations, nothing alters the validity of the concept of Calories In = Calories Out.

MYTHS

There are people with heart disease, kidney disease, and liver disease who suffer from water retention. Some medications can also cause water retention, which can result in some weight gain. We call this condition *edema*. If you think you are retaining water, you should consult your physician to see if you have any of these problems. It's also possible for people to have a very salty meal or two and experience transient water retention. This usually disappears in a day or two.

Many who claim to be overweight because of water retention are deluding themselves. This misconception permits them to perpetuate a myth and avoid dealing with the problem: *They're eating more calories than they're burning.* Some of us eat more than we admit, even to ourselves; and many of us eat more than we realize.

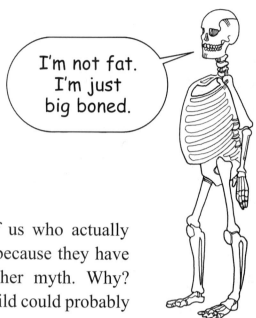

I'm not fat. I'm just big boned.

There are also those of us who actually believe they weigh more because they have "big bones." That's another myth. Why? Because a five-year-old child could probably lift your entire skeleton.

AGE AND GLANDULAR CONDITIONS

As we age, our muscle mass decreases, our activity decreases, and the rate at which we burn calories decreases. At the age of 70, most of us have a decrease in our basal metabolic rate of about ten percent. Clearly, this could result in weight gain. Other conditions, such as a thyroid hormone deficiency, can also decrease the basal metabolic rate and cause weight gain. This can usually be treated rather easily with thyroid hormone. On the other hand, an overactive thyroid gland can increase our metabolic rate and result in weight loss. Such conditions can easily be diagnosed and treated by doctors, but they are beyond the scope of this discussion.

OTHER FACTORS

Add to this the fact that some of us have poor dental structures and many of us may have developed poor dietary habits over several decades. Others may be taking medications that compromise their appetite. It's easy to see how various factors can conspire to create malnutrition. Many depressed people eat as a way of rewarding themselves and feeling more comfortable. But depression can work both ways. While depressive disorders can result in massive obesity, in still other instances, they can dampen the appetite and cause severe weight loss and malnutrition.

When you consider all possible factors, however, it still comes down to Calories In = Calories Out. *Ultimately, you are what you eat.* I know some of you are thinking that if we are what we eat, then maybe we should all go out and eat something very, very rich; cute, but not a good idea.

RESTING METABOLIC RATE

The resting metabolic rate, or RMR, is the number of calories a person would burn if he or she was at rest all day. An individual's RMR can be estimated by multiplying his or her body weight by a factor of 10. As an example: A person weighing 150 pounds probably has an RMR of about 1,500 calories a day. But this is just an approximation. Illness, fever, exposure to cold, increased digestive demands, and the like can profoundly impact the RMR. Also, when we are active we utilize even more energy. We burn more calories

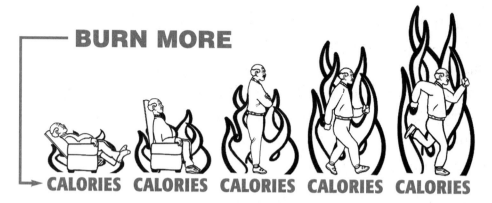

BURN MORE

CALORIES CALORIES CALORIES CALORIES CALORIES

sitting than lying down; we burn more calories standing than sitting; we burn more walking than standing; we burn more running than walking, and so on.

The upshot is that the total number of calories we burn equals the calories we burn as a result of our RMR *plus* the calories we burn as a result of activity. If, each day, we burn the same number of calories that we eat, our weight won't change. If we burn more calories than we eat, we will lose weight. If we eat more calories than we burn, we will gain weight. It's that simple: Calories In = Calories Out.

Some people just naturally burn more calories than other people. As already explained, some of that difference might have to do with the metabolic pathways. But some of it also has to do with our body makeup.

Here's an example: Even at rest, a pound of muscle burns almost 50 calories a day, while a pound of fat burns only 2 calories a day. So the more muscle and the less fat you have in your body, the more calories you burn—even at rest. In other words, your resting metabolic rate of burning calories (your

RMR) is higher—not to mention the fact that having more muscle and less fat enables you to comfortably increase your daily activity, your exercise, and your endurance. In light of this, it's clear that knowing your RMR and your body fat ratio is important to weight management. This knowledge enables you to develop your personalized dietary intake and exercise program more intelligently.

IDEAL WEIGHT AND BODY FAT

Another example: Three pounds of muscle can burn 4,500 calories a month. So adding three pounds of muscle means that you could lose about 15 pounds a year without changing your diet at all. Also, the greater our muscle mass, the more activities we can enjoy and the more calories we can burn by taking part in these activities.

Body fat, however, is not the enemy. In fact, it's important. We all need it. It helps regulate our body temperature; it serves as a storage depot of energy; it cushions our joints and protects our vital organs; it stores vitamins; and it's also used to make hormones. So some fat in our diets, particularly those that contain the so-called *essential fatty acids*, is vital to good health. What we don't need is too much body fat. An excess of body fat is associated with diabetes, high cholesterol, heart disease, hypertension, and even cancer. The upshot? *Within reasonable parameters, achieving the proper ratio of body fat to muscle is more important than achieving our ideal weight.*

Weight Ranges
(IN POUNDS)

HEIGHT IN FEET & INCHES	MINIMUM FOR ALL ADULTS (BMI=20)	RECOMMENDED MAXIMUM FOR AGES UP TO 25 YEARS	RECOMMENDED MAXIMUM FOR AGES BETWEEN 25 & 45 YEARS	MAXIMUM FOR ALL ADULTS (45+) (BMI=25)	HEIGHT IN FEET & INCHES	MINIMUM FOR ALL ADULTS (BMI=20)	RECOMMENDED MAXIMUM FOR AGES UP TO 25 YEARS	RECOMMENDED MAXIMUM FOR AGES BETWEEN 25 & 45 YEARS	MAXIMUM FOR ALL ADULTS (45+) (BMI=25)
4′9″	92	106	111	115	5′7″	127	147	153	159
4′10″	95	110	115	119	5′8″	131	151	158	164
4′11″	99	114	119	124	5′9″	135	155	162	169
5′0″	102	118	123	128	5′10″	139	160	167	174
5′1″	106	121	127	132	5′11″	143	165	172	179
5′2″	109	125	131	136	6′0″	147	169	177	184
5′3″	113	130	135	141	6′1″	151	174	182	189
5′4″	116	134	140	145	6′2″	155	179	187	194
5′5″	120	138	144	150	6′3″	160	184	192	200
5′6″	124	142	148	155	6′4″	164	189	197	205

The ideal weight chart above (adjusted for height, gender, and age) can serve as one of the guidelines for good health. However, if you weigh 20 percent more than your ideal weight, your risk of death or disease does *not* appear to be significantly greater than someone who is at their ideal weight. These ideal weights only serve as a rough assumption of the muscle-to-fat ratio in our bodies. But since appropriate muscle-to-fat ratio is important to your health, a more accurate determination of your body composition is needed. One of the most widely used methods of estimating such body composition is the determination of *body mass index,* often referred to as the *BMI.*

BODY COMPOSITION AND BMI

For those of you who like mathematics, calculating your BMI is a good way to get an understanding of your body composition.

It indicates whether or not you should be classified as obese or are otherwise at increased risk for cardiovascular complications. You can do it with pencil and paper, but it's much easier if you have a calculator—especially if you're as bad at math as I am. If you can measure your height and weigh yourself in metric units, it's also much easier. If you can't, you'll have to convert inches to meters and pounds to kilograms. The formula to calculate your BMI is simple: Divide your weight in kilograms by the square of your height in meters (kg/m^2).

George A. Bray, M.D., has simplified this calculation by developing a nomogram (page 72) that can help you determine your BMI in three easy steps. Note that the chart has three columns. Body weight, in pounds and kilograms, is in the column on the left. Height, in inches and centimeters, is in the column on the right; and the BMI is in the middle column. First, identify your weight in pounds or in kilograms and put one end of a straight edge or ruler on the body weight line at that level. Second, identify your height in inches or in centimeters and put the other end of your straight edge or ruler on the height line at that level. Your BMI can then be found in the middle column—at the point where the straight edge or ruler intersects the BMI line.

While those of us with a BMI greater than 30 are classified as obese, the risk of cardiovascular disease and diabetes progressively increases at BMI levels above 25. *That's why I believe that all of us should strive to have a BMI of 25 or less.* If your BMI is higher, you're probably eating too many drippy grilled cheese sandwiches and not getting enough exercise!

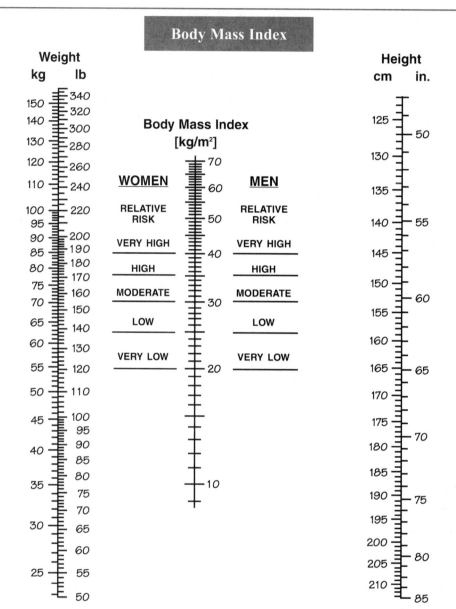

Nomogram for determining body mass index. To use this nomogram, place a ruler or other straight edge between the body weight (without clothes) in kilograms or pounds located on the left-hand line and the height (without shoes) in centimeters or in inches located on the right-hand line. The body mass index is read from the middle of the scale and is in metric units. (*Copyright 1978, George A. Bray, MD. Used with permission.*)

OTHER WAYS OF MEASURING BODY FAT

The most accurate way to determine your percentage of body fat requires a DEXA scan (see page 152) or an elaborate device that weighs you in a water bath. These services are available in some health centers. Some folks use special skin-fold calipers that measure your fat content by pinching your skin and underlying fat at different locations. I call them *pinch-an-inch* devices and have no serious confidence in their accuracy.

The distribution of body fat does appear to have substantial implications in regard to obesity-related morbidity, however. Many of the more important complications of obesity are linked to upper-body fat. Specifically, intra-abdominal obesity and abdominal wall fat (the potbelly) are associated with a greater frequency of morbidity than lower-body fat—fat on the buttocks and thighs. One can easily make the distinction by measuring your waist and your hips with a tape measure. A waist-to-hip ratio of greater than 0.9 in females or greater than 1.0 in males is indicative of excessive upper abdominal fat—and a further increase in the risk of obesity-related morbidity. Consistency is important. Be aware that fluctuations in abdominal gaseous distension, the levels at which you apply the tape measure, and the amount of tension you apply to it can affect the accuracy of these measurements.

For those of you who want an easier way of measuring your body fat, there are several affordable handheld devices on the market that can give you a reasonably accurate gauge. They work through infrared technology and can be purchased at most sporting goods stores. Bathroom scales that use bio-electric technology are also available to measure your weight, your percentage of body fat, your skeletal muscle-mass, and also calculate your RMR and BMI. While these instruments may not be as exquisitely accurate, they're a convenient and affordable way of establishing a baseline so you can monitor your progress.

It isn't essential that you use one of these devices. If you eat a healthful diet, monitor your weight, and get the proper exercise, you *will* decrease your body fat, increase your muscle mass, and take inches off in all the right places. If possible, however, I urge you to splurge and buy one of these convenient devices. *Decreasing your percentage of body fat while approaching your ideal weight is much more important than simply achieving your ideal weight.*

While many professional athletes and bodybuilders maintain body fat levels of 5 to 15 percent, that's a lot lower than I'd suggest for most of us. In my opinion, adult women should ideally have a body fat range of 20 to 35 percent. Men's body fat should be between 15 to 20 percent or even as much as 25 percent as they pass their sixtieth birthday.Take a look at the chart on the next page for a finer breakdown based on age.

COUNTING CALORIES OR COUNTING POUNDS

While we might recommend that the average-sized adult male eat 2,500 calories a day and the average female eat 2,000 calories a day, these recommendations can't apply to everyone. That could be perfect for the person who burns 2,500 or 2,000 calories a day

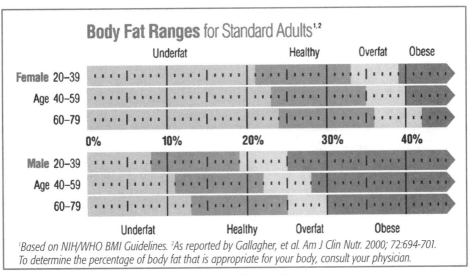

Body Fat Ranges for Standard Adults[1,2]

and who has a body fat content in the range of 20 percent. If you burn more calories, you can eat more calories to maintain your body weight and your fat ratio. If your body weight and fat ratio are higher than they should be, you have to eat less and burn more by increasing your activity and your time spent exercising.

Eating and exercising sensibly has the cumulative effect of improving the metabolic pathways to more efficiently burn energy and build muscle. As this develops, you will build more muscle mass, have more energy, and improve your health. And as your percentage of body fat decreases, your vigor and strength will increase right along with it.

Remember: If you eat even a mere 100 calories more than you burn each day, you can gain as much as 10 pounds in a year! It's important to have a general idea of your daily intake of calories. But actually counting the calories and grams of everything you eat is so difficult for most people that it causes them to fail. Within reason, you don't have to count calories—but you do have to weigh yourself. That's exactly what I want you to do. I want you to estimate the calories you take in and estimate the calories you burn by weighing yourself.

Your estimates will become increasingly accurate and fine-tuned by weighing yourself each day. That's where the rubber hits the road. If you weigh more today than you weighed yesterday, you simply ate more calories yesterday than you burned. The solution? You must take corrective action and burn more calories today than you eat today. This may mean that you have to add an extra 15 minutes to your walking or workout schedule and eat a little less for a few days, but it works! You can teach yourself to increase lean muscle and lose that extra fat without plotting your menus down to the last calorie. In this context, calories are your friends, not your enemies.

I know that some psychologists and dieticians say you shouldn't weigh yourself every day. Why? Because you'll get discouraged and depressed if you haven't lost weight. But I call that the ostrich syndrome: You bury your head in the sand so you don't know what's working and what's not. Ten days later you might find out that you gained five pounds by miscounting calories or counting the wrong calories. There's no getting around it: *You have to eat less and burn more.* The effect may be immediate or it may take a few days, but it will happen for you. You'll lose weight. Remember: Calories In = Calories Out. Every day is a new experience. Unless you're the ostrich, you're in control.

WEIGHING YOURSELF

Daily weight may fluctuate for quite some time until your caloric expenditure and your newly improved metabolic pathways have been conditioned. After that, a daily weigh-in will become increasingly valuable as a guide to your performance. Take note, however: It will be important for you to have a good scale and to weigh yourself at the same time of day, each and every day, without clothing, and after or before your morning toilet. *Consistency is most important.* Most bathroom scales are spring scales. If you are using a spring scale, your posture and the position of your feet on the scale can affect the reading by as much as three pounds or even more! Be certain that the position of your feet and your posture are the same from day to day. Consistency counts.

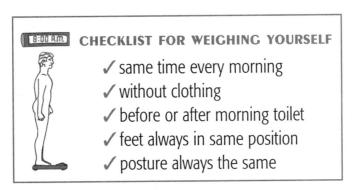

8:00 A.M. CHECKLIST FOR WEIGHING YOURSELF
- ✓ same time every morning
- ✓ without clothing
- ✓ before or after morning toilet
- ✓ feet always in same position
- ✓ posture always the same

CALORIES VS. EXERCISE

There are about 3,500 calories in a pound of fat, and a one-mile walk burns about 100 calories. So, theoretically, you would have to walk 35 miles to lose a pound of fat! If you view this in a narrow sense, you'd have to wonder why you should exercise at all. What's the point? On the other hand, if you ate 200 calories less and burned 150 calories more, you would lose a pound of fat every ten days. If you ate 500 calories less and burned an extra 500 calories a day, you would lose two pounds of fat every week.

Exercise is important for many reasons. If you lose weight without adding muscle, you may weigh less—but you might not be much healthier. Some studies have shown that obese men who are physically fit have greater longevity than men of normal weight who are not physically fit. This doesn't mean that being obese is good. Obesity has many health risks. However, the study does underscore the value of exercise and physical fitness.

Some weight loss—especially when it happens very rapidly— may actually be the loss of muscle mass as well as fat. As previously discussed, muscle tissue burns more calories than fat tissue—even at rest. So, a far healthier and more effective program is to balance calorie intake with calorie burning by exercise and muscle-building. As your muscle mass increases, you will be able to eat more calories. Actually, you may need even *more* calories to stay in balance. So the object of eating just enough to build lean muscle and improve physical performance is the ideal balance.

MENUS AND RECIPES

In terms of specific menus, there are numerous diet books, recipe books, cookbooks, and lists of menus available that have been around for years. Some of them are full of helpful ideas—but all of them are useless unless you have a solid understanding of nutrition and your own metabolism. Once you do, these diet and recipe books can be of real service. Knowing how our metabolism, our genetics, our eating habits, and our exercise habits interact will enable us to better apply the simple concept of Calories In = Calories Out.

LOOKING BACK, LOOKING FORWARD

CHAPTER 5 REVIEW . . .

◆ Calories not burned by exercise become fat stored throughout the body in fat depots.

◆ Since a gram of fat contains twice the calories of a gram of protein or carbohydrate, much more exercise is required to burn off a gram of fat.

◆ Through exercise, your metabolic pathways can become more efficient at building muscle and utilizing energy.

◆ Achieving proper muscle-to-fat ratio is more important than achieving ideal weight.

CHAPTER 6 PREVIEW . . .

◆ Why is it so important to understand the *reasons behind* lifestyle modifications in order to make a lasting commitment?

◆ Why are proteins and high-fiber carbohydrates so much healthier than fats and low-fiber carbohydrates? Are all sugars and fats bad for us?

◆ Is it possible to devise an effective program of lifestyle and nutritional change tailored to my personal tastes and goals?

6

GROANS, GRUMBLES, AND GASES

Diet cures more than lancet.
—Anonymous

Indigestion is charged by God with enforcing morality on the stomach.
—Victor Hugo

Undoubtedly, many of us have a long history of bad dietary habits that need to be altered. But most importantly, in your effort to embark on a program of healthful weight management—please avoid fad diets. Many of them work well for a time but have long-term drawbacks. Most are based on the assumption that you won't exercise in order to burn more calories and increase your muscle mass. Others seem to be based on the principle that if it tastes good, you should spit it out! If you really want to be Nifty after Fifty, it is likely that you will have to change some of your eating habits—and you definitely *will* have to exercise. But it is also important that your nutritional intake is in keeping with your individual tastes—or you won't stick with any changes made.

Modifying your diet may be more difficult for some than for others. But keep in mind that your tastes have changed over the years. You may well find some dietary changes enjoyable after you try them. It's not uncommon for people who have given up red meat for a period of time to find the taste downright disagreeable when they give it another try. While change for the better is always desirable, change of any kind is commonly viewed as difficult. That's why it's so important to understand the reasons why significant lifestyle modifications are worth the effort. In this chapter, we will learn how to fashion our own nutritional program.

FAD DIETS: LOW-CARB AND LOW-FAT

Many weight-reduction programs manipulate metabolic pathways to get short-term weight loss. Some rely on strict abstinence from carbohydrates and the development of ketosis to burn fat. Others are based on different forms of voodoo such as "low-fat" or "no-fat" snacks that are loaded with low-fiber carbohydrates. But because such snacks are low in fat as well as in fiber, they're not very satisfying or filling—so we tend to overeat them. And of course those carbs turn to sugar and then to fat. *But not all carbs are bad guys.* Aside from being filling, high-fiber carbs are also an abundant source of very important nutrients, vitamins, and antioxidants. You should also beware of "sugar substitute" snacks on the market. Why? They often contain artery-clogging fats.

Let's remember that the overall aim of weight management is to make us *healthier*. Low-carb diets, crash starvation diets, grapefruit diets, or virtually any other fad diet may cause very rapid weight loss—but that doesn't necessarily make you healthier.

THE PLEASURES OF EATING AND POSITIVE COMMITMENT

For most of us, eating is one of life's great pleasures—and I believe it should stay that way. How is that possible? For many, relying on willpower to avoid certain foods—foods that we really enjoy—has been less than effective in changing our bad eating habits. This is because we are attempting to use willpower in a negative way. I'm talking about the negative willpower that says, "Don't eat this" and "Don't eat that."

The power of positive commitment (willpower directed at what we *should* eat) tends to be much more effective. Let's take the guy who likes to eat two or three doughnuts with his coffee every morning. Instead of telling himself that he can't eat those doughnuts, suppose he tells himself that he can. But *first* he must eat a bowl of high-fiber cereal or an eggwhite omelet with high-fiber vegetables, some whole-wheat toast, and a glass of low-fat milk. Once he's fortified with healthy food, instead of eating two doughnuts he may eat one, or just a bite, or hopefully none. He was already satisfied before he even looked at a doughnut. The important decision he made was not to avoid doughnuts; it was to eat the right foods.

Some may perceive this approach as an oversimplification, but it isn't. It's real. *The change in paradigm or viewpoint is what works.* Use your willpower to eat something that's good for you. Try it. If you eat enough of the right foods in a balanced diet, you may find that you want a smaller piece of pie, or just a bite, or none at all. Your knowledge that the pie is full of fat and low-fiber carbohydrates (that will be converted to fat), backed up by your sense of satiety, may well dampen your level of desire. What you must be sure to do is to eat *enough* of the good stuff. Don't train yourself to leave room for the pie!

Another good example of how to conquer a bad habit: Many of us have long ago given up the idea of eating any breakfast at all. But a nutritious breakfast is an important metabolic kick for good health and weight management. Most of us will recall that in childhood our mothers made sure we had a nutritious breakfast before we left for school. Chances are you did that for your own children. *So why shouldn't you start doing it for yourself?* If you suspect that this will require some commitment on your part—I agree with you. That's the commitment I want you to make—to do something good for yourself that you're not doing now.

THE BALANCED DIET

A helpful guideline is the food pyramid developed by the United States Department of Agriculture. Many authorities think that even the newest guidelines are too high in sugars and fat. So keep that in mind and try to go even lower on fats and sugars. Also note that when the food pyramid was revised in 2005, an exercise category was added.

Portion size has become a "growing problem" in America. Sparked by competition, restaurants and many fast-food establishments have greatly increased portion size over the last two decades. Hamburgers are larger, portions of French fries have doubled, and soft drinks have become gigantic. The

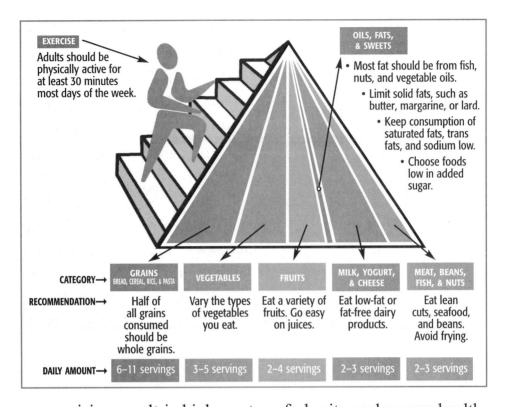

EXERCISE
Adults should be physically active for at least 30 minutes most days of the week.

OILS, FATS, & SWEETS
- Most fat should be from fish, nuts, and vegetable oils.
  - Limit solid fats, such as butter, margarine, or lard.
    - Keep consumption of saturated fats, trans fats, and sodium low.
      - Choose foods low in added sugar.

CATEGORY →	GRAINS BREAD, CEREAL, RICE, & PASTA	VEGETABLES	FRUITS	MILK, YOGURT, & CHEESE	MEAT, BEANS, FISH, & NUTS
RECOMMENDATION →	Half of all grains consumed should be whole grains.	Vary the types of vegetables you eat.	Eat a variety of fruits. Go easy on juices.	Eat low-fat or fat-free dairy products.	Eat lean cuts, seafood, and beans. Avoid frying.
DAILY AMOUNT →	6–11 servings	3–5 servings	2–4 servings	2–3 servings	2–3 servings

unsurprising result is higher rates of obesity and poorer health. Sometimes this situation is further complicated by our misunderstanding of what is meant by a serving. When trying to construct a balanced diet that suits your needs, it is important to avoid over-sizing your portions in any of the various food categories. Look at the serving size chart on the next page for some examples of reasonable portions.

Again, I'm not going to suggest menus or recipes. There are plenty of books full of delicious recipes and interesting menus. If you incorporate these ideas into your guidelines, you will be eating a balanced diet.

What is "a serving"?

GRAINS

1 slice bread

1/2 cup cooked rice or pasta

1/2 cup cooked cereal

1 cup ready-to-eat cereal

VEGETABLES

1/2 cup chopped raw or cooked vegetables

1 cup leafy raw vegetables

FRUITS

1 piece of fruit

1 melon wedge

3/4 cup fruit juice

1/2 cup canned fruit

1/4 cup dried fruit

MILK, YOGURT, AND CHEESE

1 cup milk or yogurt

1-1/2 to 2 ounces cheese

Example: A 1-inch cube of hard cheese weighs about 1/2 ounce.

Note: Buy low-fat or skim dairy products to avoid harmful fats.

Note: Some people have trouble digesting lactose, the sugar in milk products. If you have this problem, try eating yogurt with active cultures, low-fat cheese, or lactose-reduced milk. Pills and drops that help you digest lactose are also available.

MEAT, POULTRY, FISH, DRY BEANS, EGGS, AND NUTS

1/2 cup of cooked beans, 1 egg, or 2 tablespoons of peanut butter make up 1/3 of a serving of this food group.

2-1/2 to 3 ounces of cooked lean meat, poultry, or fish make up one serving of this food group.

Example: A slice of cooked, lean meat or poultry that is about 1/4-inch thick and measures 3 inches by 4 inches weighs about 2 ounces; a cooked, lean hamburger patty that weighs 3 ounces is about 3 inches across and 1/2-inch thick—about the size of a large mayonnaise jar lid.

Note: Before cooking, a patty this size weighs about 4 ounces.

Note: Half of a skinless, cooked chicken breast weighs about 3 ounces.

Note: Egg whites are a good source of protein, but egg yolks are high in fat and cholesterol. Consider discarding the yolk.

Note: Nuts are a good source of protein, but are high in fat.

FATS, OILS, AND SWEETS

The fewer fats, oils, and sweets you eat, the better.

But what if your tastes are such that you feel you must deviate from these guidelines? Try to deviate in favor of high-fiber carbohydrates and protein and against animal fats and low-fiber carbs. High-fiber carbs and proteins produce a more protracted sense of satiety. Also, proteins are absorbed more slowly than starches and sugars. That means they provide a steadier flow of energy instead of the roller coaster swings that occur from eating sugars.

Remember: When you eat starches or sugars your blood sugar goes up, and then your insulin secretion goes up to manage the surge in blood glucose (the glycemic effect). When the surge in blood glucose is brought down by the insulin surge, you eat more starches or sugar. That's the roller coaster effect—up and down and up and down again. This vicious cycle can be avoided with a diet rich in protein and high fiber carbohydrates.

THE IMPORTANCE OF PROTEINS

You will recall that there are four calories of energy in each gram of protein. Proteins in our food are the building blocks of tissue protein. When we eat proteins, our digestive tract breaks them down into amino acids for the purpose of absorption. After these amino acids are absorbed, they are reconstituted into many kinds of tissue protein. By an utterly magnificent process, protein becomes the material that makes up our muscles—the muscle tissue in our arms, legs, and back. Tissue protein makes up the facial muscles that enable us to smile or frown and the muscles in our mouths and throats that allow us to swallow and to speak. All of these are the so-called *somatic* muscles—the muscles that make up the musculoskeletal system.

The muscle tissue in the heart and in the walls of our blood vessels pumps and circulates the blood throughout our body. The muscles in the walls of the intestinal tract propel our food and nutrients in the process of digestion and excretion. These are the muscles of our viscera, and they, too, are made up of tissue protein. The importance of protein—the material that makes up our muscles—can hardly be overstated.

COMPLETE PROTEINS AND ESSENTIAL AMINO ACIDS

There are complete proteins and incomplete proteins. Complete proteins contain all of the essential amino acids; incomplete proteins contain some, but not all, of the essential amino acids. The eight essential amino acids necessary for building healthy tissue are *leucine, isoleucine, methionine, valine, phenylalanine, lysine, tryptophan,* and *threonine.* If you're going to take a protein supplement, checking a list of these amino acids might help you determine the quality of the supplement. Eggs (particularly the whites of eggs), milk, and animal protein are the best sources of these high-quality, complete proteins. The proteins in most vegetables are incomplete. Why? Because they don't contain all of the essential amino acids. So if you're a vegetarian who wants to get most of your proteins from vegetables, you must be sure to have a mixed and varied diet of vegetables, grains, and legumes to get all of the essential amino acids.

The recommended daily intake of protein varies with a person's age, gender, and muscle mass. Protein requirements are higher during adolescence than during adulthood—and they're also higher during pregnancy and lactation. People with a large muscle mass, as well as those who are exercising and building muscle, need more protein than people with a smaller amount of muscle mass.

Many authorities believe the average adult should eat 45 to 65 grams of protein a day. Others feel that 30 percent of your total daily caloric intake should be in the form of protein. For example, if you are eating a 2,000-calorie diet, 600 calories might be consumed in the form of protein-rich foods (fish, chicken, turkey, etc.). Since there are four calories in each gram of protein, that could amount to about 150 grams a day. Many, however, are concerned about a diet that is *too* high in protein—particularly in individuals with kidney or liver problems. It's true that too much protein can sometimes be hard for these organs to handle. Nonetheless, I believe that, in normal people, the danger of eating too much protein has been overexaggerated. Most people with normally functioning kidneys and a normal liver can handle the recommended amounts of protein without any difficulty. People with kidney disease or advanced liver disease—as well as people with risk factors for kidney disease such as heart disease, hypertension, or diabetes—should check with their doctor to determine how much protein is appropriate for them.

There are some additional notes of caution: You should eat a balanced diet of protein, carbohydrates, and some fat. If the proportion of your daily calories is too high in protein and too low in carbohydrates, your body can't utilize all that protein to build tissue protein. Some will be stored as fat or glycogen—or the body will try to use the excess protein for energy by converting it into sugar—but it won't be an efficient source of ready energy.

Also, if you eat too many calories at one time, even in the form of lean healthy protein, the excess calories that aren't burned will be stored as glycogen or fat. That's one of the problems experienced by those who eat one meal a day or who eat most of their total daily calories at one meal. And it's a very good reason to distribute the calories you eat over three—or even four—servings a day.

HIGH-PROTEIN FOODS
Beef and pork

Traditionally, meat has been a popular source of protein in our diets. In recent years, however, a great deal of concern has been raised about the dangers of eating red meat. On one hand, beef products can contain a lot of animal fat, which raises your blood fat and cholesterol levels. This is particularly true when you eat a greasy hamburger at some burger joint where only the Great Spirit knows what's in it. On the other hand, lean red meat—and I emphasize the word *lean*—is less than 10 percent fat and very high in protein. Lean cuts of top sirloin, flank, shank, top round, or chuck are relatively low in fat and contain about the same amount of cholesterol as skinned chicken breast. Such meats can be an excellent source of protein. Likewise, lean cuts of venison and buffalo meat are a good source of protein and are also low in saturated fat and high in essential fatty acids. Lean pork—and I don't mean spareribs; I mean lean pork—is lower in fat than most cuts of beef and is also abundant in protein. While many people cite moral issues regarding veal products, it should be noted that veal is a rich source of protein. It is lower in fat than red meat—if it isn't breaded and fried or smothered in creamy cheese or buttery sauces.

Poultry

Because the white meat in chicken and turkey breast is low in fat and cholesterol, it's one of the best choices of complete or whole-food protein. The skin of these birds, however, is high in fat and cholesterol. So it's important to remove the skin and avoid deep-fried preparations that add fat. Ground turkey and chicken burgers can be healthy if they're made of breast meat. Ground poultry often contains dark meat and skin, however. So be sure to check it out and know what you're eating.

Fish

Fish may win the grand prize as possibly the best source of animal protein. Salmon, tuna, swordfish, halibut, and most other coldwater fish are not only high in protein but also contain large amounts of essential fatty acids. They can actually *encourage* fat burning. Eating fish three times a week will probably provide you with all the necessary amounts of essential fatty acids you need and also those special omega-3 oils that appear to prevent cardiovascular disease.

It is important to avoid adding saturated fat to your fish. So avoid deep-fried preparations or sauces that smother the fish with buttery dressings. Some chefs and cooks seem to specialize in changing a healthful food like fish into an artery-clogging sea monster! On the other hand, baked, grilled, or pan-blackened fish served with salsa or some other low-fat preparation can be absolutely delicious.

Shellfish contain a substance called *sterols* which were once thought to cause high cholesterol. While some authorities believe this to be exaggerated, others claim you can get 100-plus milligrams of cholesterol in a single serving of shellfish. Shellfish, such as lobster and crab, are high in protein. But again, avoid fried preparations and the creamy butter sauces that are so commonly served with them—or you will be adding a lot of saturated fat to your diet.

Non-meat protein foods

Non-meat foods such as low-fat cottage cheese and eggwhites—or some of the commercially prepared products made of eggwhites—are chock-full of protein. More than just low in calories and a good source of protein, eggwhites make excellent omelets with the addition of onions, spinach, mushrooms, and salsa. Did you know that many highly competitive athletes eat no meat at all? They get all of their proteins from low-fat dairy products, eggwhites, and vegetables.

Aside from any moral issues that might relate to eating meat, consider the economics of feeding the world's population: Cattle walk, run, grow, and burn calories. Cattle must be fed about 20 calories of grain to produce one calorie of beef! That's why there are so many people who contend that raising beef to please our palates is a wasteful use of our planet's resources. Lentils, soybean products, chickpeas, lima beans, navy beans, black-eyed peas, and many other such foods are loaded with nutritious proteins.

Recent studies have also suggested that eating beans three times a week may decrease your chances of having a heart attack by as much as 19 percent. (Obviously, I don't mean refried beans; they're usually loaded with cholesterol and saturated fat.) One cup of beans contains almost 15 grams of protein. While I'm not suggesting that you have to be a vegetarian to be healthy, there's no doubt that, if you choose to do so, you can satisfy all of your protein requirements without meat.

VEGETABLES, DAIRY PRODUCTS, AND GASEOUSNESS

Many vegetables—and particularly beans—produce intestinal gas. To a great extent, this reaction decreases after a few weeks of eating these foods. Why? Your intestinal tract simply becomes more adept at handling them. Also, a product on the market called *Beano* (which can be sprinkled on the beans) tends to reduce the gas formation. People who have a lot of allergies, such as an allergy to penicillin, can be allergic to Beano—so it's not recommended for them. Your pharmacist, however, can recommend one of the silicon products on the market that may decrease gaseous distension by defoaming the gas (breaking up the bubbles). This allows the gas to diffuse throughout your intestinal tract more easily. Tablets containing charcoal (a potent absorbent of gas) can also be useful. If gaseousness after eating beans or vegetables is a continuing problem for you, ask your doctor for further recommendations.

For those of you who like to cook, special ways of preparing beans can also reduce gas formation. Soaking the dried beans for eight hours, slow cooking, and adding a little baking soda, some tomatoes, and citric acid seems to reduce the gas produced by beans.

LACTOSE INTOLERANCE

The most likely cause of gaseous distension following the ingestion of milk products is *lactose intolerance.* Produced in the upper part of our intestines, an enzyme called *lactase* is responsible for digesting *lactose*, which is the sugar present in milk products. When there is a deficiency in this enzyme, the lactose is not properly digested, so it subsequently undergoes fermentation, resulting in excessive gaseous distension. "Colicky" infants occasionally have this problem and are given milk substitutes. Babies usually outgrow colic by developing the ability to produce sufficient intestinal lactase to comfortably drink milk and eat milk products.

Lactose intolerance is usually a benign disturbance that is very common in otherwise healthy adults. Sometimes, however, it is associated with inflammatory bowel disease. There are several diagnostic tests to prove the diagnosis of lactose intolerance, but, in my experience, the simplest test is to temporarily stop the ingestion of milk products (milk, ice cream, cheese, etc.) and see if the gaseous symptoms disappear.

Most often, the situation is easily managed by limiting the ingestion of milk products or by using milk from which the lactose has been removed, and fortunately, lactose-free milk or milk with reduced lactose is available at most grocery stores. You can also purchase lactase supplements. These tablets, which can be taken prior to ingesting lactose-rich products, seem to significantly reduce gaseousness in many people.

CARBOHYDRATES

Beans, along with other vegetables and fruits, are an excellent source of carbohydrates because they also contain important vitamins, antioxidants, and fiber. It's important to remember, however, that simple sugars and refined starches such as white rice and mashed potatoes are carbohydrates that become blood glucose: If you don't burn 'em, they will turn to fat.

Because carbohydrates are such an important source of energy, *I recommend that about 40 to 60 percent of your total daily calories consist of complex carbohydrates such as beans, fruits, and green vegetables.* These foods contain soluble and insoluble fiber, which supports the health of your intestinal tract.

"SWEET" MYTHS

Fructose, also known as *levulose*, is the sugar in fruits. It's a great source of energy—but please understand that it's *sugar* and quickly converts to glycogen. (So if you don't burn it, you know what it becomes!) Remember that glycogen is the starch stored in your muscles and your liver. So it's another case of *Burn* or *Blubber*.

Eating fruit is healthy because it furnishes your body with vitamins, fiber, and antioxidants, but don't delude yourself with the popularized myth that fructose has a magical quality—it's sugar. If you gorge yourself on fruit, you can get fat. So get the amount of fruit in your diet suggested by the food pyramid, but make vegetables your primary source of complex carbohydrates. Like fruit, vegetables are high in fiber and vitamins, but unlike fruit, they are low in sugar.

Brown sugar and honey require special mention. Sugar is sugar is sugar. The sugar in brown sugar is *sucrose*, the same as in white sugar. Whether it's brown or white, it's converted to glucose. And in regard to honey, note the following: Plants and flowers produce a thick, viscous substance containing sucrose, the same sugar that's in white or brown sugar. That's what the bees harvest. This is converted to fructose and glucose.

Athletes believe honey to be a good source of energy for two reasons: The glucose provides immediate energy, and the fructose can be readily stored as glycogen to provide a more delayed source of energy. But don't harbor any myths—it's still sugar. The choice is yours: *You either pump up and burn it, or you don't, and blubber up.*

Sugar is a good source of quick energy. But again, it's important that you get most of your carbohydrates in the form of complex carbs that are high in fiber and important nutrients.

FATS

As previously stated, there are nine calories in every gram of fat—more than twice the number of calories in proteins and carbohydrates. It's no secret that fat can clog up your arteries and result in heart attacks and strokes. But not all fat is bad. The major fat culprits are found in red meat, the so-called *saturated fats.* Most of the fats found in vegetables are *unsaturated* fats such as the polyunsaturated fats and monounsaturated fats found in guacamole and macadamia nuts. They're the good guys. The unsaturated fats in vegetables may actually help lower your blood triglycerides and cholesterol and protect you against heart disease. Olive oil, sesame oil, canola oil, and safflower oil are examples of such beneficial fats.

Physical wellbeing requires essential fatty acids in your diet for nutrition as well as for digestive purposes. Vitamins A, D, E, and K are fat-soluble vitamins. These vitamins, along with some other important nutrients called *carotenoids,* do not dissolve in water but are soluble in fat. So some fat in your diet is required to absorb these nutrients. *Lycopene*, for example, is the red carotenoid found in tomatoes and watermelon. It's currently being studied as a possible weapon against prostate and other cancers. *Lutein* is another example that's found in green vegetables and has been linked to heart health and eyesight. *Beta *carotene,* found in carrots and cantaloupe, and *zeaxanthin,* found in corn, are still other fat-soluble nutrients.

Recent studies have revealed that adding some avocado to a salad can increase the absorption of lycopene (more than four times), beta carotene (more than two times), and lutein (more than seven times). In a similar vein, the nutrients from a bowl of cereal and berries are likely to be better absorbed using 2% milk than skim milk.

For salads, choosing heart-healthy unsaturated fats such as those in avocado and olive oil would seem a healthier choice than nonfat salad dressings. If the nutrients you eat don't get absorbed, what good are they? On the other hand, don't forget that fats have nine calories per gram—more than twice the amount that proteins and carbohydrates have. So try having your salad dressing served on the side—and limit the amount you use by dipping your fork.

It's also important to note that some fats from the vegetable world are dangerous and should be avoided. Coconut oil and palm oil, for example, are highly saturated, and hydrogenated oils contain unhealthy trans fats that may actually slow the absorption of good nutrients and clog your arteries. Some artificial creamers contain these oils.

I recommend that on a daily basis, no more than 30 percent of your calories come from fat. Moreover, it would be wise to keep your intake of saturated fat (animal fat) lower than 10 percent of your daily calories.

CHOLESTEROL

Cholesterol is important because the body uses it to produce hormones and cell membranes. The cholesterol in your blood is derived from two basic sources: the cholesterol you eat and the cholesterol your liver manufactures. It seems likely that your genes determine and control the amount of cholesterol your liver makes. Some people's livers make very little cholesterol—so they can gorge themselves on high-cholesterol food and still have normal blood levels. All of us can think of someone we know who can eat bacon, eggs, steak, ice cream, and chocolates in large amounts every day and never have a cholesterol problem. Other people can severely restrict their cholesterol intake but still have high blood cholesterol because their liver makes so much. When cholesterol blood level gets too high, it can accumulate on the walls of our arteries and cause heart attacks and strokes.

Egg yolks and dairy products such as milk, butter, cheese, and ice cream are examples of high-cholesterol foods. Red meat, the skin on chicken and turkey, and the dark meat of these birds contain more cholesterol than you need. Organ meats such as liver, brain, pancreas, and thymus gland are also high in cholesterol, as are some shellfish. So a low-cholesterol diet is one that restricts these foods—one that is low in dairy products, red meat, and egg yolks and high in fish, the white meat of chicken and turkey, fruits, and vegetables.

It may surprise you to know that many studies suggest that younger people are at much greater risk from elevated blood cholesterol levels than older people. Elevated cholesterol is a major risk factor for the development of coronary artery disease and heart attacks, particularly in middle-aged men and women. Beyond middle age, high cholesterol levels appear to be less of a risk factor.

Because of this finding, it might be concluded that older people don't have to restrict their cholesterol. *I don't agree.* There is no good reason to continue a bad habit by assuming that the damage is already done. What folly to prolong a bad habit because someone else has decided it won't impact your longevity! I say it *can* affect your longevity and your vitality. Think it through. You're going to live longer than the preceding generation, and the generation following you will live longer than your generation. The so-called "middle age" period of life will be redefined. Many of the terrible effects that high cholesterol has on our blood vessels can be stayed and even reversed by a low cholesterol intake and exercise. Don't give up on yourself! *Limit your cholesterol intake to 100 mg a day.*

GOOD CHOLESTEROL AND BAD CHOLESTEROL

It's important that you know there is no so-called "good cholesterol" in the food you eat because there's no food source for good cholesterol—also known as HDL. *You can't eat good cholesterol; you have to make it.*

Let me explain. Special carriers in our blood called *lipoproteins* transport cholesterol throughout the body. The most important of these are called low-density lipoproteins or LDL (bad cholesterol), very low-density lipoproteins or VLDL (very bad cholesterol), and high-density lipoproteins or HDL (good cholesterol). For the most part, LDL is the bad cholesterol that clogs up our arteries and causes heart attacks and strokes—by eventually closing the artery off. Eating too much cholesterol is the major cause of this condition. But remember that in some people, genetics play a very important role.

So-called "good cholesterol" or HDL may actually remove bad cholesterol from the walls of the arteries and bring it to the liver, where it may be metabolized or harmlessly excreted into the bile. Exercise, weight loss, and stopping smoking can all have a very beneficial effect on increasing the levels of good cholesterol.

For good health, we like to see the total cholesterol below 150, the bad cholesterol or LDL below 130, and the good cholesterol above 30 or 35. Most of you can achieve this with diet and exercise. In cases where diet and exercise do not produce the desired effect, your doctor can prescribe cholesterol-lowering medications that have proven to be very effective.

TRIGLYCERIDES

The significance of *triglycerides*, the other fat substance that's made in the liver and circulates in our blood, is somewhat controversial. Normal levels range up to 200 milligrams. High levels appear to be a risk factor for heart attacks, particularly among women, and more recently, high triglyceride levels have been linked to an increase in the frequency of strokes.

Triglyceride levels often decrease as the good cholesterol (HDL) levels increase. A healthy diet and exercise can also be effective in decreasing your triglyceride levels.

THE HEALTHFUL DIET

A good general guideline is the "40–30–30" rule. You should get about 40 to 50 percent of your calories from carbohydrates (mostly high-fiber carbs), about 20 to 30 percent from proteins, and no more than 30 percent from fats. Try to keep the animal fat low (less than 10 percent) by avoiding the saturated fat contained in most red meat and dairy products. If you're a committed carnivore, and you feel you *must* eat red meat, try grass-fed beef or even wild game such as venison instead of the traditional grain-fed beef.

Vegetables, poultry, and fish should be your main sources of protein. A diet rich in fruits and vegetables is also rich in fiber, vitamins, minerals, and antioxidants. For example: Purple grape juice and red wine are loaded with chemicals called *flavonoids*. They can thin the blood and improve the elasticity of blood vessels. Oranges, apricots, and bananas are rich in potassium and can help lower blood pressure. Less common fruits such as pomegranates contain an enzyme called *paroxonase* that can break up the arterial plaque on our arteries.

Heart-friendly foods are higher in the polyunsaturated omega-3 oils. These oils improve the flexibility of arteries and may even reduce the inflammatory reaction of blood vessels. You can find lots of them in fish, canola oil, walnuts, and flaxseed.

Hydrogenated vegetable oils can cause serious damage. They are made of the so-called *trans fats*. These not only raise your level of LDL, the bad cholesterol, but they can also decrease your level of HDL—the good cholesterol. So limit your intake of hydrogenated vegetable oils.

The saturated fats in dairy products and red meat also raise your levels of bad cholesterol. Try to substitute them with polyunsaturated fats and the monounsaturated fats in things like avocados and olive oil. While there is no food source for HDL, some foods have the tendency to both increase your good cholesterol (HDL) and decrease your bad cholesterol. Olive oil and the organosulfurs in onions might do this. And please—*make it a habit to read the labels on the foods you buy.* Try to stay away from too many chemicals or preservatives.

MENU ADDITIONS

Some studies suggest that for men, having one or two alcoholic drinks a day, particularly red wine, is heart healthy and may actually be associated with greater longevity. Be aware, however, that men and women appear to metabolize alcohol differently. In women, recent data seems to indicate that a couple of alcoholic drinks a day may be associated with an increase in the frequency of breast cancer. But more data is needed before a final determination can be made.

Some studies suggest a beneficial effect from drinking two cups of tea a day and also eating a little chocolate—particularly dark chocolate. (This means one or two pieces of chocolate, not a boxful!) Dark chocolate, with a cacao content of 60% or more, has a greater antioxidant punch than milk chocolate.

Additional points of interest: There are now some scientific reasons to believe that fish, walnuts, asparagus, and berries—particularly blueberries—can improve or help preserve brain function. Mice that were fed blueberries, for example, dramatically improved their ability to negotiate a maze. While I suspect there's some truth in all these scientific stories, the jury is still out. But it's really interesting, isn't it? Mom always said that fish was brain food—and now there appears to be some scientific evidence that the blueberry is, too.

As you will recall, fish contain those wonderful omega-3 oils, which are great antioxidants. And it seems that the polyphenols in tea and some other foods have multiple beneficial effects. All of the above being said, don't slavishly eat the same thing every day. Vary your foods. *After all, variety is the spice of life!*

LOOKING BACK, LOOKING FORWARD

CHAPTER 6 REVIEW ◆ ◆ ◆

- ◆ Significant lifestyle changes can be achieved through positive commitment.

- ◆ The USDA food pyramid is a useful guideline for good nutrition.

- ◆ A diet rich in protein and high-fiber carbohydrates increases both energy and muscle mass.

- ◆ Limiting consumption of sugars and fats promotes heart health as well as general fitness.

CHAPTER 7 PREVIEW ◆ ◆ ◆

- ◆ What factors contribute to common excretory problems such as constipation and diarrhea?

- ◆ What's the difference between soluble- and insoluble-fiber foods? Which kind of fiber can prevent disease and benefit diabetes?

- ◆ Are there any risks in using stool softeners and laxatives regularly?

- ◆ Is it absolutely necessary to drink six to eight glasses of water a day?

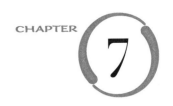

FIBER, FLUIDS, AND FECES:
A Cause-and-Effect Relationship

*Give me a good digestion, Lord,
and also something to digest.*
—A Pilgrim's Grace

*It's a very odd thing—as odd as can be—
that whatever Miss T eats . . . turns into Miss T.*
—Walter De La Mere

THE SCOOP ON POOP

What goes in must come out (particularly in the case of fiber): It's as simple as that. So let's briefly review stool formation and evacuation—a wonderment to the very young during their potty training, but sometimes a problem for older people.

Ingested food is propelled through the body by contractions of the muscles within the walls of the digestive tract. These waves of muscular contractions are called *peristalsis*. As the food passes through our stomachs and our small intestines, it is digested and the nutrients absorbed. The residual material (feces) is passed into the colon, where water is absorbed, causing the stool to solidify. This newly solidified fecal material is then moved farther along into the rectum by the peristaltic contractions of the colon.

When the amount of feces in the rectum and lower colon reaches a critical point, the urge to defecate becomes apparent.

The act of defecation is comprised of several components. It begins with a forceful bearing down as the diaphragm and the abdominal musculature contract. This causes an increase in intra-abdominal pressure. That pressure, together with increased peristalsis, is followed, almost immediately, by an exquisitely coordinated reflex in the ano-rectal area involving relaxation of the anal sphincters and elevation of the anus by a muscle called the *levator ani*. Then, under normal circumstances, the stool drops.

CONSTIPATION

Any significant change in bowel habit can signal the presence of a mechanical obstruction to the flow of the stool. This might be caused by a tumor or inflammatory narrowing. Sudden or recurrent changes—whether in the form of constipation or diarrhea—should be evaluated by a physician.

Now we know that too little dietary fiber and inadequate fluid is likely to result in constipation—a malady that tends to worsen as we age. This may take the form of straining or difficulty in passing the stool, infrequent bowel movements (less than three a week), or a feeling of incomplete evacuation. Frequent straining at stool may result in hemorrhoids, painful fissures or cracks around the anus, the development of diverticulosis, or even the extrusion of some of the rectum's lining, a condition called *rectal prolapse*—but more about some of this later.

It isn't hard to see that weakness of any of the musculature involved in defecation—or any disease process that affects the neuromuscular activity of these muscles or the intrinsic muscles of the colon—can cause constipation. As an example, weakness of the muscles in the abdomen or the pelvic floor may contribute to constipation. Also, many authorities believe that irritable bowel syndrome, a very distressing but relatively benign condition, is the result of a defect in the neuromuscular activity of the intestinal wall. This condition can cause constipation, diarrhea, or both.

Alternatively, any of the following factors might be responsible for constipation: inactivity or a lack of exercise, laxative abuse, the use of constipating medications, or the habitual postponement of the urge to defecate. The wide variety of issues that can contribute to constipation underscores the need for people with this condition to get a thorough physical examination. Your physician may recommend additional tests such as sigmoidoscopy, colonoscopy, x-rays, or perhaps even special testing, depending on the individual circumstances of your case.

The list of medications that can cause or contribute to constipation is a mile long. "Suspects" can range from antacids you might take for dyspepsia to the side effects of any medications that alter bowel activity. Narcotics and other pain relievers, some bowel-relaxing drugs called anticholinergics, and even some tranquilizers are examples. So check with your doctor if you develop constipation while taking medication.

DENYING THE URGE

We have the ability to deny the urge to defecate because the external anal sphincter is under our voluntary control. But the frequent and habitual denial of this urge is a bad idea. Why? Because it can cause chronic constipation. Prolonged retention of the stool allows more water to be absorbed, making the stool get harder. More stool entering the area and more denial causes even more hardening. When you finally go to the toilet, you grunt and groan and strain—a bad habit. If this becomes a routine, the rectum acclimates to an increased volume of hard stool and is less and less sensitive to its presence. That may delay the normal signal to evacuate—starting a vicious cycle that ends in the development of chronic constipation.

FECAL IMPACTION

Taken to the extreme, the compacted stool can become voluminous, causing what is referred to as a *fecal impaction*. Fecal impactions can fill and obstruct the rectum, requiring a visit to the emergency room where an oil retention enema followed by digital disimpaction is performed to remove the stool from the rectum—not a pleasant experience.

Among the elderly, fecal impaction is particularly common as a result of dehydration coupled with a sluggish bowel. It may also occur in hospitalized patients as a result of the inactivity imposed by bed rest and/or the use of constipating medications. The unfamiliarity of the hospital environment alone can cause a conscious or unconscious delay in defecating. That's why promptly responding to the urge, taking in adequate fluids, and staying active (regular exercise) are important tools in the prevention of constipation.

LAXATIVES AND ENEMAS

Many people seek to alleviate constipation with enemas or laxatives. While the use of these remedies to solve the occasional problem can be valuable, *the more laxatives you take, the more you need.* Why? The neuromuscular complexes responsible for normal defecation can become dependent on the stimulation produced by frequent use of laxatives and enemas. The result is that these reflexes seem to rely upon these stimulants to act. You want to avoid getting into that situation. If you're already there, however, you can try to retrain your colon by gradually tapering off laxative use and increasing your intake of fiber and water. If you must use a laxative, use the mildest one that works for you—and use it for the shortest period of time possible. That having been said, be aware that laxatives can be classified into different categories, depending on their mechanism of action. There are irritant laxatives, hyperosmolar and saline laxatives, stool softeners, and bulk-forming laxatives.

Irritant laxatives such as Dulcolax, Senokot, Ex-Lax, and Feen-A-Mint actually irritate the lining of the colon and stimulate expulsive contractions. These can be associated with cramping abdominal discomfort, loss of nutrients, and a proclivity to induce dependence.

Hyperosmolar laxatives consist of mixed-electrolyte solutions containing polyethylene glycol or nonabsorbable sugars such as lactulose or sorbitol. How do they work? They cause an outpouring of fluid into the colon that increases the pressure and liquidizes the stool. While primarily used for cleansing the bowel before diagnostic procedures, MiraLax (containing polyethylene glycol) or lactulose (a non-absorbable sugar) are occasionally prescribed in cases of severe chronic constipation.

Saline laxatives are very popular. The most commonly used is Milk of Magnesia. Like the hyperosmolar laxatives, they also work by pulling fluid into your colon to make the stool softer and easier to pass. But the frequent use of saline cathartics can cause fluid retention in the elderly—a serious problem for people with high blood pressure and kidney or cardiovascular disorders. They should not be used on a regular basis.

Stool softeners are not really purgatives. They don't actually cause you to have a bowel movement, but rather soften the stool, making it easier to pass. Although stool softeners are not harmful, be careful when you use them. They can cause you to stain your undergarments because of the occasional inadvertent passage of stool. Some popular examples are Colace, Dialose, and Surfak.

Mineral oil is *both* a laxative and a stool softener. It can lubricate the bowel and soften the stool—but it can also interfere with the absorption of nutrients, particularly the fat-soluble vitamins. It happens rarely, but people who have difficulty swallowing sometimes inhale mineral oil into their lungs, which results in a nasty condition called lipid pneumonia. For these reasons, mineral oil is best used as a retention enema to soften hard stools. When taken orally, it should be used sparingly and taken only on an empty stomach.

Bulk-forming laxatives, because they consist of some form of plant fiber, are safer than most others. Popular brands such as

Metamucil, Serutan, and Citrucel probably account for 15 to 30 percent of laxative use in the United States. These products facilitate defecation by drawing water into the colon and absorbing the water. This makes the stool softer, larger, and easier to pass. However, it's a good idea to take a full glass of water with these bulk formers to avoid hardening the stool. It's also important that they be used an hour or two after any other medications to avoid interfering with their absorption.

A note of caution regarding *high-colonic enemas:* The colon cleans itself by regenerating most of its lining every 24 to 48 hours. The rationale for a high-colonic cleansing enema (often recommended to clean out toxins) is a myth without scientific merit. In fact, this procedure has been associated with serious complications (and has more value in the treatment of *mental* constipation than anything else)!

FLUIDS

Ingesting the right amount and the right kinds of liquids, while important for many reasons, is essential in preventing chronic constipation. Fluid requirements vary from one individual to the next. Climatic conditions, a person's size, and their level of physical activity are the key determinants. The hotter and dryer the climate, and the greater our physical activity, the greater our fluid requirement will be. While we've often heard that everyone should drink six to eight glasses of water a day, I don't know the scientific basis for that recommendation. Use your common sense; if you're thirsty, drink some water. Beyond that, it's important to emphasize that hot days and physical exertion will significantly increase your fluid requirements. So under these conditions, it only makes sense to drink more water. You should be able to satisfy your fluid requirements from the food you eat and also by drinking water and healthful beverages.

Beverages containing alcohol or caffeine, such as coffee or even tea, don't count as much. *Be aware that caffeine is a diuretic, and so is alcohol.* They can cause the kidneys to work overtime and may even cause you to lose as much or more fluid than you drink. Fruit juices are a good source of fluids because they're packed with vitamins (but you *do* have to watch the calories). While drinking water is the most definitive way of making sure your fluid intake is adequate, there's lots of water in food, particularly vegetables and fruits. Drinking water is good, but drinking eight glasses of water on top of a healthful, fluid-rich diet can be a little too much—especially for some people with heart, kidney, or liver problems. These folks should check with their doctor in regard to their fluid requirements.

FIBER

Although we've all seen the TV commercials about fiber supplements, many of us don't understand what fiber actually *is*. Let me explain. The fiber in plants (vegetables and fruits) is the stuff that gives the plant its strength and its structure. It's the skeleton of the plant—that's the part of the vegetable or fruit that isn't absorbed. Most fruits and vegetables contain two kinds of fiber: *soluble fiber* and *insoluble fiber*. Both kinds benefit us in similar, but also in somewhat different ways. The difference between them is simple: Soluble fiber can dissolve in water and insoluble can't. Let's take a look at this diagram of the intestinal tract.

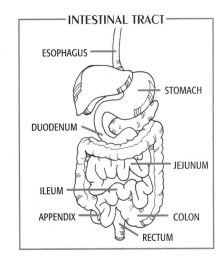

INTESTINAL TRACT

ESOPHAGUS

STOMACH

DUODENUM

JEJUNUM

ILEUM

APPENDIX

COLON

RECTUM

Insoluble fiber adds bulk to the stool in the lower intestine by absorbing water. In this way, it improves the progress of waste material through the colon. *Soluble fiber* slows the emptying time of the stomach and the motility of the small bowel. This produces an increased sense of satiety or fullness—a greater sense of satisfaction. Because of its *gelling* properties, soluble fiber also aids in the regulation of glucose absorption. Bulk formation is further increased because of soluble fiber's ability to absorb water. This improves the lubrication and transportation of waste, and it also decreases the pressure in the colon and rectum.

In addition to absorbing water and producing bulk, soluble fiber enters into a chemical reaction with the bacteria present in the human colon. This chemical reaction is a fermentation process like the kind that curdles milk or the one used to make wine. In your colon, this reaction produces fatty acids that may protect the colon from cancer and may also improve the liver's metabolism of glucose and fat. Both soluble and insoluble fiber are important—but soluble fiber seems to play a greater role in the prevention and treatment of many diseases.

THE FIBER CONTENT OF FOOD

Most high-fiber foods contain both soluble fiber and insoluble fiber. Insoluble fiber is found in nuts, dried beans, whole-grain cereals, wheat bran, and many vegetables. Soluble fiber is also found in these vegetables—as well as in oat bran and psyllium. See the table on the next page for the fiber content of some common foods. You may well find some surprises there: For example, many people assume there's a lot of fiber in lettuce, so they rely on it as a major source of fiber. In fact, however, there is comparatively very little fiber in lettuce.

The average American diet includes about 10–15 grams of fiber a day. I recommend that this be increased to about 25–30 grams a day. Using this table, you should be able to pick a lot of foods you like. At first, it may seem inconvenient to remember which foods to shop for. But I assure you that after only a couple of weeks, you'll have it down pat, and choosing high-fiber foods will become part of your new good eating repertoire.

THE BENEFITS OF FIBER

Colon tumors

Colon polyps are benign tumors of the colon—some of which may turn into colon cancer. In fact, it's believed that *most* colon cancers begin as benign polyps. A lot of solid scientific evidence shows that dietary fiber reduces the development of polyps (which should also reduce the occurrence of colon cancer).

Some very well-done studies, however, have recently shown that a high-fiber diet, taken over four years, did not prevent

FIBER CONTENT (IN GRAMS) OF SELECTED FOODS

Item	Size/Serving	CONTENT PER SERVING Soluble Fiber	CONTENT PER SERVING Insoluble Fiber	CONTENT PER SERVING Total Fiber
FRUITS & NUTS				
Almonds (roasted)	1/2 cup	0.78	7.17	7.95
Apple (with peel)	1 medium	0.97	1.79	2.76
Apricots	1 cup	1.25	2.18	3.43
Banana	1 medium	0.64	1.55	2.19
Cantaloupe	1 wedge	0.64	0.43	1.07
Grapefruit	1 medium	2.21	1.4	3.61
Grapes	1 cup	0.34	0.78	1.12
Orange	1 medium	1.9	1.19	3.09
Peanuts	1/2 cup	2.38	3.96	6.34
Pear (with peel)	1 medium	1	3.32	4.32
Plums	1 medium	0.66	0.33	0.99
Prunes (canned)	1 cup	7.88	5.88	13.76
Raspberries	1 cup	0.49	5.79	6.28
Strawberries	1 cup	1.04	2.83	3.87
Walnuts	1/4 cup	1.4	0.9	2.3
Watermelon	1 slice	0.96	0.96	1.92
BREADS, CEREALS, & OTHERS				
Bread – Rye	1 slice	0.36	1.35	1.71
– White	1 slice	0.24	0.25	0.49
– Whole-wheat	1 slice	0.46	1.65	2.11
Cereal – Bran	1 ounce	1.45	7.27	8.72
– Corn flakes	1 ounce	0.1	0.35	0.45
– Oat bran	1 ounce	2.04	2.13	4.17
– Oatmeal (cooked)	1 ounce	1	1.5	2.5
– Shredded wheat	1 ounce	0.45	2.18	2.63
Rice (cooked) – Brown	1/2 cup	0.37	4.9	5.27
– White	1/2 cup	0.31	1.11	1.42
Spaghetti	2 ounces	1.47	1.09	2.56
VEGETABLES				
Asparagus	1/2 cup	0.31	1.17	1.48
Broccoli	1/2 cup	1.15	1.42	2.57
Brussels sprouts	1/2 cup	1.41	2.09	3.5
Cabbage, green	1/2 cup	0.56	0.95	1.51
Carrots	1/2 cup	0.94	1.48	2.42
Cauliflower	1/2 cup	0.77	1.54	2.31
Celery (raw)	1/2 cup	0.42	0.54	0.96
Corn	1/2 cup	1.31	1.72	3.03
Cucumber	1/2 cup	0.1	0.42	0.52
Green peas	1/2 cup	0.48	3.04	3.52
Green string beans (canned)	1/2 cup	0.46	1.43	1.89
Kidney beans	1/2 cup	1.38	4.1	5.48
Lettuce, iceberg (raw)	1 cup	0.1	0.7	0.8
Lima beans	1/2 cup	0.85	3.57	4.42
Onions (raw)	1/2 cup	0.64	0.64	1.28
Pinto beans	1/2 cup	1.86	4.09	5.95
Potato (baked w/skin)	1 medium	0.7	0.78	1.48
Spinach	1/2 cup	0.47	1.61	2.08
Tomato (raw)	1 medium	0.45	0.72	1.17
White beans	1/2 cup	1.06	3.67	4.73

recurrent polyps during that four-year period. That said, I would emphasize the word *recurrent*. These patients had polyps previously, which suggests that they either had a genetic proclivity to develop polyps or they might have already done dietary damage to their colons by not eating enough fiber in prior years. And here's something else to consider: Because the study was conducted over a four-year period, it doesn't mean that a high fiber intake wouldn't have prevented the frequency of recurrent polyps over a longer period of time—say, 20 years.

On the flip side, many observational studies strongly suggest that a high-fiber diet is protective against developing colon tumors. In certain parts of the world (such as Africa and Asia) where most people's diets are high in fiber, colon tumors are very uncommon. It has also been observed that when Asians and Africans immigrate to our country and adopt our low-fiber dietary habits, their frequency of colon tumors begins to increase until it approximates the overall incidence seen in America. There is still much to be learned on this subject. Whether you believe that fiber protects you from colon tumors or not, there are still plenty of good reasons to eat a high-fiber diet. Let's get into some of them now.

Hemorrhoids and diverticulosis

We know that fiber absorbs water, lubricates the stool, and promotes or enhances peristalsis—the propulsive motor activity of the colon. In this way, fiber decreases the internal pressures in the colon and rectum. The result is that the development of hemorrhoids and diverticulosis are also decreased. Here's why:

HEMORRHOIDS

Normally, we have these little anal cushions filled with tiny blood vessels in our rectum—down near the anus. As the pressure in the rectum increases, the shearing force on these anal cushions also increases. Over a protracted period of time, the increased shearing force causes the supporting tissues around

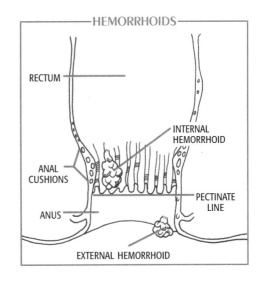

these little anal cushions to become progressively weaker and to develop into hemorrhoids. As the pressure continues, the hemorrhoids get larger and larger—and more engorged with blood. And as the supporting structures become weaker and weaker, the hemorrhoids continue to enlarge—and perhaps may even prolapse or telescope downward and protrude out the anus. After a bowel movement some people have to actually push their hemorrhoids back up with their fingers. Sometimes the condition progresses to the extent that the hemorrhoids get stuck and *can't* be pushed back—so surgery is required. When hemorrhoids enlarge, their covering tissue gets stretched, causing the hemorrhoids to become painful, itch, or bleed.

Study the illustration above. Notice that the last part of the anus is lined by tissue similar to skin. The upper part of the anus and rectum is lined by tissue similar to that of the colon. The line that divides upper from lower is called the *pectinate line*.

A hemorrhoid that develops above this line is called an *internal hemorrhoid*. If it develops below the line, it's called an *external hemorrhoid*. Since an external hemorrhoid is covered by skin-like tissue, it can itch and become very painful. Sometimes, a blood clot forms inside the hemorrhoid which requires surgical evacuation. Because of this, external hemorrhoids can be very painful, but also, because of this thick covering of skin, they usually don't bleed.

On the other hand, internal hemorrhoids (formed above the pectinate line) are covered by the same kind of lining as the colon. This is a thinner covering that has few or no pain nerves. So internal hemorrhoids have a greater tendency to bleed—very often without causing any pain or discomfort. A high-fiber diet and a good fluid intake can decrease the internal pressure in the colon and rectum. And when we decrease the pressure, we decrease the shearing force. The result? Hemorrhoids can often be reduced in severity or even prevented.

DIVERTICULOSIS

Diverticulosis is characterized by the development of small pouches or pockets at weak points in the colon. Most physicians believe that low-fiber diets are primarily responsible for causing diverticulosis. A diet low in fiber increases the internal pressure in the colon and causes the muscles

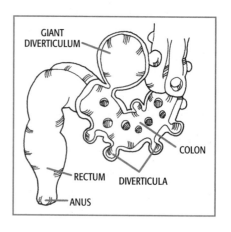

in the colon's wall to strain and get thicker. Weak spots then develop between these thickened bands of muscle. Under increased internal pressure, the weak spots in the colon tend to bulge outward and form pockets, or *diverticula*.

Diverticulosis became most evident at about the same time that refined flour and other processed foods were introduced in the early 1900s. (Whole-wheat flour contains an abundance of bran, whereas refined flour has no wheat bran at all.) It's significant that diverticulosis is most prevalent in well-developed, industrialized population groups such as those in the United States and England. This ailment is not problematic in the less-developed countries of Asia and Africa—where diets are higher in fiber content.

Diverticulosis is often asymptomatic. Sometimes, however, it's associated with bloating and constipation, along with mild to moderate abdominal discomfort and cramping. Bleeding, sometimes quite severe, can also occur. This bleeding is believed to come from the rupture of tiny, weakened blood vessels in a diverticulum. While the bleeding usually stops on its own, on rare occasions it can be life threatening. At that point blood transfusions or surgery may be necessary.

What happens when these pockets or pouches become infected and inflamed? A condition called *diverticulitis* is created. (It's *diverticulosis* when there is no inflammation or infection, and *diverticulitis* when there is.) Diverticulitis can be a very serious problem. Usually the infection can be cleared up in a few days with antibiotics. Sometimes, however, an abscess forms or an infected diverticulum perforates like a ruptured appendix. When this happens, pus spills into the abdomen, causes peritonitis, and surgery is often required. Given the all-too-real risks, it's clear that we're well-advised to follow a high-fiber diet in order to prevent the development or progression of diverticulosis. The best way to eliminate any possibility of these miserable complications is to avoid the problem in the first place by eating enough fiber.

Fiber and diabetes

Soluble fiber slows the emptying of your stomach. That produces a sense of satiety or satisfaction, which in turn makes it easier for you to eat less, lose weight, and follow your diabetic diet. Also, the gelling action of soluble fiber smooths out the absorption of carbs and sugars. This decreases the roller coaster ride (the glycemic effect) of high sugar—high insulin—lower sugar—eat more sugar—high insulin—and more fat formation. The smoothing effect on the absorption of carbohydrates can also benefit diabetes.

Fiber and fat absorption

Soluble fiber can also reduce the absorption of fat and cholesterol. That's very good news, because it helps lower your cholesterol and reduce your chances of getting a heart attack. All of us should take in about 25 to 30 grams of fiber a day. If you don't get enough of it in your food (vegetables, fruits, nuts, or oat bran), ask your doctor. He or she might recommend psyllium or some other fiber supplement.

LOOKING BACK, LOOKING FORWARD

CHAPTER 7 REVIEW • • •

◆ A diet rich in high-fiber foods decreases the incidence of constipation, diverticulitis, hemorrhoids, and possibly polyps of the colon.

◆ We should strive to eat 25–30 grams of fiber daily.

◆ Soluble fiber benefits diabetes and helps to lower cholesterol.

◆ Laxatives should be taken sparingly; the more you take, the more you need.

◆ Fluid requirements vary and are affected by climatic conditions and physical exertion.

◆ Caffeinated beverages and alcohol are diuretics; by making your kidneys work overtime, too much can cause you to lose as much fluid as you drink.

CHAPTER 8 PREVIEW • • •

◆ Does our need for various vitamins and minerals change as we age? Are herbal supplements beneficial?

◆ Are synthetic vitamins as good for us as the natural vitamins we get in vitamin-rich foods?

◆ What are the best dietary sources of important beta carotene and lycopene?

8

VITAMINS, ANTIOXIDANTS, HERBS, MINERALS, AND OTHER SUPPLEMENTS

*Life expectancy would grow by leaps and bounds
if green vegetables smelled as good as bacon.*

–Doug Larson

A vitamin is a substance that makes you ill if you don't eat it.

–Albert Szent-Gyorgyi

DIETARY SUPPLEMENTS

For many years physicians were taught that a nutritious diet made dietary supplements unnecessary. It was believed that a healthful diet contained enough vitamins and minerals. Taking extra vitamins, we were told, had the effect of producing expensive urine—but did not add to health! In other words, the body would use what it needed and the rest would be excreted in the urine—or perhaps not even absorbed but passed in the stool. At that time conventional medical wisdom actually condemned the use of supplemental vitamins except in cases of vitamin deficiencies caused by such things as starvation, inborn errors in absorption or metabolism, and disease states associated with wasting or interference in the absorption or utilization of nutrients.

To a large extent, the pendulum has now swung in an equally inappropriate direction. These days it's commonplace for people to gulp a handful of vitamins and herbs on a daily basis. People do this in the sincere belief that these pills and powders will improve their memory, their strength, and their potency— not to mention their longevity! *This is the result of clever marketing.* The ad writers have convinced a lot of us that we need these expensive supplements to restore strength and youthful energy.

The fact is that the ingredients in many of the items touted at fancy health-food stores can be purchased at a drugstore for a fraction of the price. Moreover, the safety and the value of many of these supplements are questionable. Why? Because they don't fall under the province of FDA evaluation. That's why false claims, based on less than adequate scientific study, can be made so blithely. Worse than mere exaggerating, some of these products may actually be harmful. Still other supplements—that would normally be harmless—might interfere with the action of certain medications. So check with your doctor before taking any of these herbs or supplements. Don't part with your money too quickly!

As a result of accumulating scientific information, conventional wisdom is changing in favor of taking certain supplements—but definitely *not* megadoses of vitamins or a whole handful of herbs each day! You should get most of your vitamins from a balanced daily diet and use supplemental vitamins and minerals only when truly needed. A few examples: Some of us are on crazy fad diets to lose weight, and some of us just don't eat right. Some of these fad diets don't give us enough fresh vegetables, fruits, and fish. In the name of healthful weight loss, we may unwittingly deprive ourselves of important nutrients (omega 3 fatty acids, antioxidants, vitamins and minerals, etc.). Under these conditions, I suggest you consult with your physician or a good dietician. Taking selected vitamin and mineral supplements is an alternative way to address some of these issues.

ANTIOXIDANTS

Let's begin with a discussion about free radicals and antioxidants. What are they? Free radicals cause cell damage. For this reason, they have been dubbed the "agents of aging" in that they cause us to "rust," so to speak—in much the same way that free oxygen radicals in the air cause iron to rust. These free radicals have been linked to many diseases such as cancer, cardiovascular disease, cataracts—maybe even wrinkles—and a host of other degenerative phenomena. Our natural defense against these culprits appears to weaken with advancing age, stress, and disease.

Antioxidants act as free radical vacuum cleaners—they're our most effective weapons against these damaging substances. Fruits, vegetables, and fish are loaded with antioxidants—as are certain vitamin and mineral supplements. But it's always possible to get *too* much of a good thing, isn't it? So it's important to know just how much of these vitamins, minerals, and other supplements we *should* be getting and how much might be harmful.

VITAMIN A, BETA-CAROTENE, AND LYCOPENE

These three antioxidants seem to be very important for our immune systems and our vision. Beta-carotene, the precursor of vitamin A, is converted to vitamin A by a self-limiting metabolic process. Carrots, dark green leafy vegetables, and fish are excellent sources of beta-carotene and vitamin A—as are eggs, milk, and liver.

How much of these vitamins might be *too* much? The habitual and excessive ingestion of carrots can impart a yellowish discoloration to the skin called *carotenemia*. Outside of causing skin discoloration, however, this is usually a benign condition. A similarly harmless discoloration has been noted in some people from a chronic overindulgence in tomatoes. Tomatoes contain a pigmented substance called lycopene, another good antioxidant. Don't let this information prevent you from eating tomatoes or carrots, however. They're very healthful—and you have to eat a lot of them to develop these conditions—which disappear when you stop overindulging!

However, excessive ingestion of vitamin A can cause serious problems. Because this vitamin is easily absorbed and tends to accumulate in the liver, caution should be exercised. If toxicity occurs, it can cause diarrhea, nausea, dizziness, and drowsiness. In the long term, overdosage can even cause enlargement of the liver and spleen. Some of the members of an expedition to the North Pole are a good example. They became seriously ill from eating polar bear liver—which, unbeknownst to them, had an extremely high concentration of vitamin A.

Many multivitamin preparations contain 3,000 to even 5,000 International Units (IU) of vitamin A per tablet. This, added to the fact that many of our foods are supplemented with vitamin A, is too much. Recent studies suggest that this amount of vitamin A might actually encourage the development of osteoporosis. *So watch your dosage.* Read the labels and don't take more than 2,000 IU (0.7 mg) for women or 2,800 IU (0.9 mg) for men.

VITAMIN B12, FOLIC ACID, AND VITAMIN B6

With advancing age, the lining of the gastrointestinal tract can get thin and begin to wear out. When this occurs in the stomach, the condition is called *atrophic gastritis*. It's often associated with a decrease in the absorption of B12 and folic acid. Leafy vegetables, fruits, and yeast are good sources of folic acid or folate. But if your ability to absorb folate decreases, you still might not be getting enough. Even normal blood levels, or blood levels on the low side of normal, have been associated with serious health problems such as strokes and heart attacks. Some studies suggest these deficiencies may also be associated with dementia.

About five percent of us will also develop a B12 deficiency as we get older. Vitamin B12 deficiency can lead to anemia (pernicious anemia) and serious nerve damage. Folic acid can mask the anemia caused by B12 deficiency, but it won't prevent the nerve damage. That's why you shouldn't take folic acid without also taking B12. The two are neatly combined in many of the commercially available multivitamin preparations at your drug store.

HOMOCYSTEINE, FOLIC ACID, AND VITAMIN B6

For quite some time, doctors have been aware of an increased risk of heart attacks, strokes, and a multitude of other conditions associated with atherosclerosis in people who have an elevated level of an amino acid called *homocysteine*. The vascular changes associated with elevated levels might account for the declining mental abilities observed in some of these patients. In addition to increasing the likelihood of vascular dementia, some recent studies have indicated that even small elevations in homocysteine levels may increase the chance of getting Alzheimer's disease by as much as 40 percent.

Homocysteine levels are found to be higher in men than in women, and they tend to increase with age. Higher levels are found in cigarette smokers, people with high blood pressure and high cholesterol, and people who simply don't exercise enough.

A rare genetic disorder can also cause elevated levels of homocysteine in children. Children and young adults afflicted with this disorder suffer from severe vascular disease. All this evidence seems to indicate that an elevated level of homocysteine is definitely not good.

Vitamin B6 and folic acid can help prevent elevated homocysteine levels. Some studies have shown that people with diets high in B6 and folic acid have a decreased risk of developing heart disease, but it has not yet been established that taking supplements has the same beneficial effect. There's lots of B6 and folic acid in chicken and fish—and to a lesser extent in oats, wheat, and nuts. Garlic is also believed to decrease homocysteine levels. (But if you eat too much of it, you may become unpopular with your friends!)

VITAMIN C

Vitamin C, also known as *ascorbic acid*, is an important antioxidant. Severe deficiency causes scurvy. Milder deficiency has been linked to a variety of other conditions including heart disease, easy bruising, poor wound healing, cancer, and memory loss.

The support for these claims is less than definitive. But even *less* definitive is the belief that vitamin C can prevent colds or other viral illnesses. A brilliant, non-physician Nobel laureate believed that taking vitamin C would prevent colds—so he recommended taking 500 mg or more a day. Some people began to take 1,000 mg and even 2,000 mg a day as the idea became more and more popular. Yet in spite of many enthusiastic vitamin C advocates, numerous scientifically performed studies have dispelled the myth that vitamin C prevents colds or even shortens the course of a cold. It should also be noted that there have been no scientifically performed studies to the contrary.

A recent scientific study is of even greater concern. It suggested that taking more than 500 mg of vitamin C each day might cause thickening of the coronary arteries. Larger doses may cause diarrhea and kidney stones. As I've already stated, we must remember that *too much of a good thing can be harmful*. Multivitamin preparations usually contain 60 mg of vitamin C, which is 100 percent of your recommended daily allowance (RDA). And you also get plenty of vitamin C from citrus fruits, tomatoes, potatoes, and berries.

VITAMIN D

Vitamin D is quite another story. Milk, butter, eggs, fortified cereals, and seafood are all good food sources of vitamin D. Exposure to the sun is also important; sunlight actually helps our body produce vitamin D. But we're also told that exposure to the sun is largely responsible for skin aging, skin cancer, and the development of melanoma. Because of this, the authorities who urge us to limit our exposure to the sun are quite correct. But if a lack of sunlight is coupled with a poor dietary intake, vitamin D deficiency can develop. This sequence of events is common in people who are institutionalized, and also occurs in the homebound elderly.

The importance of vitamin D is that it increases the utilization and absorption of calcium. As we will discover in the next chapter, *this is extremely important in making and maintaining strong bones and in decreasing age-related bone loss.* In the past, we believed that 400 IU of vitamin D was the appropriate daily requirement. Now, however, studies have shown that some people have low blood levels of vitamin D despite that intake—and that bone fractures are more common in those people. Because of these findings, most doctors have come to recommend that the daily intake of vitamin D be increased to 700 or even 800 International Units. Most multivitamin pills have about 400 IU in each pill, and many supplemental calcium pills have vitamin D added to them. Women and older men need about 1,200 mg of calcium a day, and most diets have only about 700 mg to 800 mg a day—so supplements of vitamin D and calcium are important. We'll talk more about this later.

VITAMIN E

There appears to be good evidence that vitamin E, another important antioxidant, is beneficial in promoting cardiovascular health, strengthening the immune system, and possibly even improving prostate health. But the exact amount to take each day is controversial. While toxicity is an unlikely event, some studies suggest that taking more than 200 to 400 International Units a day may actually be associated with an increase in cardiovascular events. Until further research settles this controversy, I would suggest you try to get most of your vitamin E from a healthy diet. Green leafy vegetables, nuts, vegetable oils, and wheat germ are all good food sources of vitamin E. If you're going to take vitamin E supplements, I recommend that you limit it to 200 IU per day.

On another note, the difference in the value of natural vs. synthetic vitamin preparations is usually unimportant, but this may not be the case with vitamin E. Many experts believe that natural vitamin E may be much better utilized by the body than synthetic preparations—another good reason for getting most of it from your diet. Vitamin E is also known as *tocopherol,* of which there are different kinds. Synthetic vitamin E consists almost entirely of alpha-tocopherol, whereas natural vitamin E is a mix of alpha-, gamma-, and delta-tocopherols. Many experts believe that gamma-tocopherol plays a more important antioxidant role than previously suspected. So if you're going to take a supplement, check the label carefully. Natural vitamin E is labeled *Natural,* but sometimes things are labeled "Natural" when they're really not. If you're not sure, ask the pharmacist.

VITAMIN K

Green leafy vegetables are a good source of vitamin K. Smaller amounts are found in eggs, meat, and dairy products. Vitamin K plays an important role in our blood-clotting mechanism. The bacteria that are normally present in our colon are important in furnishing our vitamin K requirements. This vitamin is *not* added to multivitamin tablets because deficiency of vitamin K is extremely rare. One of the exceptions is when it is caused by certain antibiotics—which knocks out the bacteria in our colon that make vitamin K. In this uncommon situation, your doctor might prescribe a brief course of treatment with a vitamin K supplement.

FAT-SOLUBLE VITAMINS

Simply stated, "fat-soluble vitamins" are vitamins that are soluble in fat. Remember my description of the difference between soluble and insoluble fiber? I indicated that soluble fiber is fiber that is soluble in water. Well, fat-soluble vitamins are vitamins that are soluble in fat. Because of that, they're easily stored in our fat tissue and also in our liver. Most importantly, since they're soluble in fat, they're probably better absorbed after eating a meal that has some fat. Many of us take our vitamins before breakfast, so perhaps we're not absorbing all that we could. Vitamin A, vitamin D, vitamin E, and vitamin K are the so-called fat-soluble vitamins—that's A, D, E, and K.

IRON

Iron is a very important mineral. One of its most important functions is the role it plays in making *hemoglobin*, the essential part of our red blood cells. When these red blood cells are pumped through our lungs, the hemoglobin picks up the oxygen we inhale and carries it to the muscles and all of our body tissues. It's important that we have enough iron to make enough hemoglobin. If not, we develop *anemia*, which means we have fewer red blood cells than we're supposed to have. There are many kinds of anemia and other causes for it, but this kind is called *iron-deficiency anemia*. In this case, we not only have fewer red blood cells, but the blood cells themselves are smaller and contain less hemoglobin than they should. As a result, they can't carry as much oxygen to our body parts—which may make us weak and easily fatigued.

Meat, vegetables, fortified cereals, and eggs are excellent sources of iron. Most of us get all the iron we need from these foods. Many people, however, take lots of iron pills and syrups to improve their energy level or to combat fatigue. I'm opposed to this practice for two reasons. First—it can mask the presence of an iron-deficiency problem that may be of a serious nature. Second—in some people, iron can accumulate in the liver and worsen or actually *cause* liver disease. It's true that the symptoms of iron-deficiency anemia can be quickly corrected by taking iron—but that isn't always good news. Although sometimes the result of poor nutrition or impaired absorption, *iron-deficiency anemia is often caused by chronic blood loss*. A number of conditions, ranging from the very benign to the very serious, can be responsible for this. Typical examples: peptic ulcer disease, colon cancer, colon polyps, hemorrhoids, and excessive menstrual bleeding—just to name a few.

Any kind of chronic blood loss can drain your iron stores and cause iron deficiency and anemia. And because a small but continued blood loss can be protracted over a long period of time, an individual might be unaware of it until he or she develops anemia along with the symptoms of weakness and fatigability. If these symptoms are treated by taking iron pills—*without determining the cause of the iron-deficiency anemia*—the consequences can be serious. To avoid masking a significant condition, never take iron pills or supplements without your doctor's knowledge or recommendation.

SELENIUM

Chicken, fish, nuts, and vegetables are good sources of a mineral called *selenium*—another important antioxidant. Brazil nuts, tuna fish, and asparagus are particularly rich in this mineral, although it is also found in bread and meat. Many studies have strongly suggested that this mineral-antioxidant has cancer prevention qualities. For example, in areas where there are high levels of selenium in the soil, there appears to be a lower rate of death due to cancer. Other studies have shown a decrease in lung, prostate, and colon cancer in people taking a supplement of 200 micrograms (mcg) a day. Most multivitamin preparations contain about 20 mcg of selenium. If further scientific studies confirm the value of larger doses, it is likely that the amount of selenium in multivitamin preparations will be increased in the future. Until then, enjoy the benefit of a healthy intake of fish, vegetables, poultry, and nuts—but stay alert to the calories in nuts. Although Brazil nuts are particularly high in selenium, don't go *too* nuts about nuts!

ZINC AND OTHER MINERALS

A host of important minerals and trace elements are part of our body makeup. Examples include selenium and iron, which we've already discussed. Zinc, magnesium, manganese, chromium, and molybdenum are among many others. For the most part, in the United States, deficiencies in these minerals are extremely rare. We get sufficient amounts in our diet. Green leafy vegetables, fruits, whole grains, and lean meats serve as generous sources of these microelements. Additional supplementation doesn't appear to be necessary and could actually be harmful.

Zinc deficiency has been linked to diminished sexual performance and an altered sense of taste and smell. In the most unusual and extremely rare circumstance of severe zinc deficiency, enlargement of the liver and spleen and the development of anemia have been reported. Note, however, that the daily requirement of zinc is about 15 mg. This is the same amount contained in most multivitamin pills. And you also get plenty of zinc in a healthful diet. So I don't see any logical reason to take any more.

CHROMIUM

Some advocates have suggested that chromium is a "fat burner," and that taking chromium supplements can help a person lose weight and build muscle. But I don't buy it. Studies have shown no difference in weight loss or muscle development between groups taking chromium and those taking a placebo (a sugar pill). I would not recommend chromium as an additional supplement until some solid research proves it to be beneficial.

CALCIUM

Calcium, along with vitamin D, is extremely important to bone health. As you know, vitamin D plays an essential role in the utilization of calcium. Dairy products, foods that are fortified with calcium, and vegetables such as broccoli and kale are rich dietary sources of calcium. Older adults need about 1,200 mg to 1,600 mg of calcium and about 700 IU to 800 IU of vitamin D daily. Many of us get only about 700 mg of calcium in our diets and, as previously discussed, an insufficient amount of vitamin D. So taking calcium with vitamin D supplements is a good way to slow or help prevent the bone loss that accompanies osteoporosis. Tablets containing 500 mg to 600 mg of calcium with 400 IU of vitamin D are available without a prescription. Since vitamin D is fat soluble, better absorption is likely to be achieved by taking one tablet after breakfast and one after dinner.

Potentially excessive calcium can cause the accumulation of calcium crystals in the kidney. These crystals can coalesce to form kidney stones. This appears less likely to occur when using calcium citrate tablets. Why? Because citrate, in physiological concentrations, can help prevent the formation of these calculi. It must be noted, however, that some people have a pronounced tendency to form calcium kidney stones. Their condition may be worsened by taking calcium.

There are also people who have an uncommon hormonal problem known as *hyperparathyroidism* and people who have certain kinds of cancer that can elevate the level of blood calcium. These conditions can increase the proclivity to form kidney stones—more good reasons to be certain that your doctor is aware of all of your supplements.

HERBS

The study of herbs has given rise to many important discoveries—and doubtless there will be many more in the future. Heart medications such as digitalis and pain relievers derived from opium are obvious examples. Herbal remedies have been used for centuries, and undoubtedly some of these herbs are effective—but many are not. These days it's popular to take herbs to improve your memory, the health of your prostate, your sexuality, and your immune system. *I say, lots of luck!*

Your need for any of these herbs should be thoroughly discussed with your doctor. The important thing is to produce maximum benefit while minimizing the risk of doing harm. While it's true that it often takes 10 years for a scientific discovery or theory to get to the point of public consumption, *please be careful.* Although many herbs may be of benefit, some may be harmful to you. Some *so-called* scientific claims are not so scientific. If the benefits of taking something are not clearly and scientifically demonstrated, and the risks of taking it have not been thoroughly evaluated, I urge you not take it.

Fair warning: Some dietary supplements that *sound* like herbs actually contain raw animal parts. A bottle labeled "thymus" may contain bovine lymphoid tissue rather than the herb thyme. The term *orchis* can be easily mistaken for a plant herb instead of an extract from the testicle of a bull. In one instance, extracts from 17 different bovine organs (including ingredients from spleen, brain, lymph glands, and pituitary glands) were found in a supplement.

Don't be taken in. Shouldn't these labels be legible without a magnifying glass? And shouldn't the list of ingredients be descriptive? Still more disconcerting, these ingredients may be imported from foreign countries and susceptible to all kinds of contamination, including the agents that cause mad cow disease.

Presently, the Department of Agriculture's ban on these imported substances applies only to those that are to be used in food and medicines—and *not* to those to be used in dietary supplements. This is a catastrophe waiting to happen. Again, if the risks *and* the benefits of taking something are not firmly and scientifically established, please don't take it until you've consulted your doctor. Remember that eating a healthful diet will provide you with a very substantial and safe intake of nutrients.

DHEA

The letters *DHEA* stand for a long chemical name—dehydroepiandrosterone. Health food stores throughout the country have promoted DHEA as a virtual fountain of youth. It's been touted as the answer to a multitude of aging problems that range from preventing cancer, osteoporosis, diabetes, and cardiovascular disease to improving sexual performance and the immune system. Some people have even promoted it as an anti-dementia substance.

The fact is that DHEA is a hormone that's normally produced by the adrenal glands and then converted by the body into estrogen and testosterone. Because the production of DHEA decreases as we get older, proponents believe that taking it can increase our blood levels to approximate the levels found in younger adults.

Although DHEA may in fact have some health benefits for certain individuals, more animal research followed by human research is needed to determine the proper dose, the actual benefits, and the risks or side effects. Presently, we don't know if it's good—or who it's good or not good for. For one thing, the proportion of estrogen and testosterone produced by taking DHEA is not predictable, and may well vary from one individual to the next. (One person might get too much estrogen, and another person might get too much testosterone.) We just don't know. Before we buy into all the hype, my advice is to wait for the results of some reliable scientific studies.

HUMAN GROWTH HORMONE

Human growth hormone (HGH) and a substance called *insulin-like growth factor* have been suggested as anti-aging agents. Human growth hormone is naturally made by the pituitary gland, which is located just under the surface of your brain. Several studies have demonstrated an increase in muscle mass and bone strength in older men and women given HGH. Long-term followup studies, however, revealed that many of the benefits were not maintained and some actually reversed after a period of time. Some scientists think that HGH stimulates the production of insulin-like growth factor, which may be the substance responsible for some of the observed benefits. Research in progress will hopefully determine whether any real and sustainable anti-aging benefits can occur by giving either HGH or insulin-like growth factor to

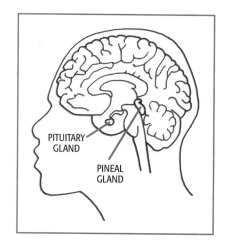

the elderly. If the research shows that the major benefits are derived from insulin-like growth factor—*and* if the cost and side effects of this kind of treatment are minimal—it could be a huge and exciting boon to anti-aging treatment. The potential side effects and the cost of treatment with HGH need to be seriously considered, however.

The excessive production of HGH is usually the result of a tumor or overactivity in the pituitary gland. When this situation occurs in adults, it can produce a condition called *acromegaly,* which is associated with unusually large hands, distortion of facial bones, and a host of other abnormalities. (A famous heavyweight boxing champion, Primo Carnera, suffered from this condition.) An excess of this hormone in childhood can cause tremendous growth and abnormal height—a condition called *giantism.* At one time some people afflicted with this condition became popular circus performers that were unkindly referred to as "freaks." Of greater concern, this condition appears to be associated with high blood pressure and early death. So, before going across the ocean or south of the border to get this kind of treatment, we must learn more about the true benefits and side effects of HGH.

MELATONIN

Melatonin is a hormone produced in the pineal gland (shown in the illustration on the previous page), which is situated deep inside the brain. This hormone appears to have antioxidant properties and may also strengthen the immune system. Higher levels are produced at night—which is one reason it seems to be important in helping us sleep. Lower levels of melatonin have been noted in the elderly as compared to the levels usually found in young adults. These low levels have been linked to the insomnia that is so common in advancing age.

Many travelers have touted melatonin as a cure for jet lag, and others have advocated it as a sleep remedy. In some individuals, small doses of 0.1 mg to 0.3 mg have been shown to improve the quality of sleep and shorten the time required to fall asleep. But larger amounts have been associated with headaches and drowsiness. Melatonin doesn't require a doctor's prescription. But be aware that the dose commonly sold in stores can be as high as 3 mg—many times the amount that seems to be needed.

However, a recent study done on blind patients started with doses as high as 10 mg a day. (Those who are blind live without many of the external environmental factors that influence sleep.) Starting with this high dose, many of the patients did experience a restoration of their normal sleep rhythm and even maintained it when the dose was gradually reduced to 0.5 mg a day. The timing of the dose was individualized in each patient as determined by blood tests that measured their natural levels of this hormone. A lot of research is still being conducted on the long-term effects of melatonin. My opinion? Taking melatonin in small amounts (1 mg) once in a while on an intermittent basis doesn't appear to be harmful—but I can't recommend it as a daily or regular supplement until we have more solid data. And I wouldn't recommend it in high doses except under the supervision of a physician.

LOOKING BACK, LOOKING FORWARD

CHAPTER 8 REVIEW ◆ ◆ ◆

◆ Too much vitamin A can damage the liver and encourage the development of osteoporosis.

◆ Supplements of vitamin D and calcium can help prevent age-related bone loss.

◆ Most vitamin and mineral supplements should be taken only when truly needed; overdoses can have serious consequences.

◆ Certain vitamins and minerals, when provided by a healthful diet, are powerful antioxidants that mitigate the damage done by free radicals.

CHAPTER 9 PREVIEW ◆ ◆ ◆

◆ Is hormone replacement therapy worth the risk?

◆ Can osteoporosis be prevented or reversed?

◆ What happens to our bones as we grow older? Is there anything we can do to help protect ourselves from fractures?

◆ Is it true that certain forms of exercise can effectively fight osteoporosis?

◆ What is osteoarthritis, and what are the most effective ways to deal with it?

HORMONE REPLACEMENT AND YOUR BONES AND JOINTS

*A man's health can be judged by which
he takes two at a time—pills or stairs.*

—Joan Welsh

The best and most efficient pharmacy is within our own system.

—Robert C. Peale

ESTROGEN

After the onset of menopause, estrogen replacement (by means of pills or patches) appears to retard the progression of osteoporosis, or what some people refer to as "softening of the bones." Why is this so important? Because it may well decrease bone fractures, bone pain, and shrinking height. Many women who take ERT (estrogen replacement therapy) have also noted a dramatic improvement in their sense of wellbeing and their quality of life. Some of the specific effects cited include control of hot flashes and night sweats, improved sexuality, smoother skin, and better vaginal lubrication. For these reasons, estrogen replacement appears to have a decided anti-aging effect.

Estrogen also appears to have a positive effect on the brain. How? By encouraging the growth of brain cells and improving their chemical activity. It's unclear whether it has any effect on people with Alzheimer's disease. Some studies indicate memory improvement, but others have failed to confirm these findings. We'll have to await the results of additional research while the stew simmers.

Despite all these wonderful benefits, however, estrogen therapy is not without risks.

Recent research has shown an increased risk of breast cancer, uterine cancer, heart attacks, and strokes in some women who take estrogen and progesterone as hormone replacement therapy (HRT) for menopause. For those who have a strong family history of these problems, the risks seem to outweigh the benefits. Despite all the perceived benefits, HRT is no longer the routine treatment it used to be. Like so many other things in life, each of us has to weigh the risk-to-benefit ratio of doing something or not doing it. So the decision to take or not take estrogen must always be individualized and thoroughly discussed with your doctor.

TESTOSTERONE

The male climacteric is the male counterpart of the female menopause. Generally, however, it occurs more gradually. During this change, there is a decline in the production of testosterone (the male sex hormone) along with a corresponding decline in libido and sexual performance. When testosterone is given to castrated men, there is marked improvement in muscle size and strength—and, in some cases, an improvement in sexuality. But in normal men the effects are less consistent.

Testosterone does not appear to improve impotence in most men. Why is this so? Because impotence appears to be related less to testosterone deficiency than to the presence of other problems such as vascular disease, diabetes, and psychological factors such as depression. It's a fact that the frequency of these problems increases with age—and also that many medications used to treat these disorders can further decrease libido and sexual performance.

Testosterone is an androgenic steroid that builds protein and muscle; that's the upside. But there's a potentially serious downside, too. It may provoke or enhance the growth of prostate cancer, and it may encourage the development of coronary artery disease, liver disease, or even male baldness and the growth of facial hair. Research on testosterone therapy and its ability to improve muscle and bone strength is ongoing. Hopefully, some answers as to its anti-aging effects will become clearer in the not too distant future. Until then, be patient and take testosterone only for specific reasons—and then only under the advice and watchful eye of your physician.

Testosterone is probably not as hazardous as some of the other anabolic-androgenic type steroids (such as the muscle- and protein-building steroids that some athletes and bodybuilders take). We've all read the horror stories about healthy athletes suffering from liver disease, liver cancer, premature heart disease, and God knows what else as a result of these steroids. Some of them do have some medical uses, but—*please* don't take them unless advised by your doctor for a specific reason.

OSTEOPOROSIS

Osteoporosis—a loss of bone mass and bone mineral density—affects both men and women. It starts earlier and is more severe in women. That's why, when we get older, many of us will get shorter and suffer serious fractures. Underscoring the devastating consequences of osteoporosis, *falls and fractures are actually a greater risk factor than obesity in the elderly.* An example: In the United States, there are about 30,000 to 35,000 deaths related to hip fractures each year—and more than 20,000 of them occur in post-menopausal women.

The anatomy of bone

How much do you know about the makeup of bone? A better understanding of your bones will help you better understand osteoporosis. Let's use a big bone like the femur, or thigh-bone, as an example. The outer portion of the bone is called *cortical bone,* and the inner or more central part of the bone is called the *matrix.* This is also known as *cancellous* or *trabecular bone.* The

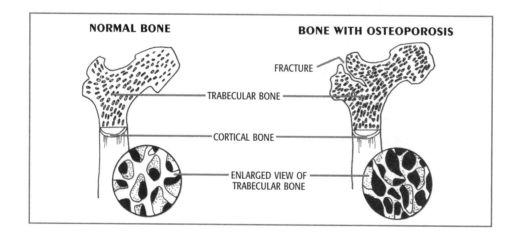

NORMAL BONE   BONE WITH OSTEOPOROSIS

FRACTURE

TRABECULAR BONE

CORTICAL BONE

ENLARGED VIEW OF TRABECULAR BONE

cortical bone is more or less solid, and the matrix or trabecular bone is sort of a honeycombed network of bone tissue.

Bone remodeling (bone production and bone loss)

The continuous remodeling of bone is a constant and very exciting process. By "remodeling" I mean that bone is in a constant state of flux. While new bone is being made, old bone is being taken away—a process called *resorption.*

This process of bone remodeling (bone production and bone resorption) continues throughout our lives. During our years of growth, new bone production occurs at a much more rapid rate than bone resorption. When we reach the age of 30 or 35, bone mass reaches its maximum. The rates of production and resorption are generally in equilibrium until we are about 40 or 50 years of age. After that, the rate of bone resorption begins to exceed the rate of bone production, and our bone mass begins to decrease.

The rate of bone loss accelerates appreciably in women around the time of menopause—when the amount of bone loss can be as high as 40 to 50 percent. Although bone loss is slower and less drastic in men, it can still be quite serious—as high as 20 to 30 percent. Loss of trabecular bone begins slightly earlier than the loss of cortical bone and is of much greater magnitude in women.

The spine and hips are usually most affected—primarily due to a loss in trabecular bone. Correspondingly, fractures involving our hips, wrists, and backs are more problematic as we age.

Vertebral bone fractures—cracks in those little bones that make up the spine—are usually *compression fractures* that cause a loss of height or even alter the curvature of the spine.

The agents of bone production are little cells known as *osteoblasts* (bone makers), and the agents of bone resorption are little cells known as *osteoclasts* (bone takers). Since the remodeling of bone is a continuing process throughout our lives, both the osteoblasts and the osteoclasts serve important functions. The osteoblast cells produce new bone, and the osteoclast cells resorb bone.

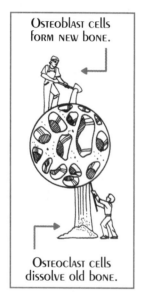

Osteoblast cells form new bone.

Osteoclast cells dissolve old bone.

Osteoblasts are extremely active during stages of growth and at the site of fractures—where they produce new bone to heal the fracture. With advancing age, the activity of the osteoclasts (the agents of bone resorption) exceeds the activity of the osteoblasts. But how do we know if we have osteoporosis or to what extent our bones have demineralized? The gold standard is a test called the DEXA scan.

DEXA scan

The term D-E-X-A is short for *dual energy x-ray absorptiometry* —DEXA. This test is not only painless, but it's also not associated with exposure to high levels of radiation. It's far more effective than conventional x-rays in determining bone density and diagnosing osteoporosis. As a screening procedure, peripheral scans rather than total body scans can be performed on the ankles or on the wrists. If the scans suggest osteoporosis, a total body scan can be performed to determine the severity and extent of the condition. People who are at high risk for osteoporosis can benefit from these screening procedures. How? The scans can encourage our use of the preventative and therapeutic measures to be discussed and also monitor the effectiveness of treatment.

Treatment and prevention

Although estrogen and testosterone deficiencies accelerate bone loss, hormone replacement therapy is reserved for exceptional cases. Because of their potential to produce harmful side effects, they are no longer part of the routine regimen against osteoporosis. Calcium and vitamin D supplementation, however, are extremely valuable and should be used in the amounts previously discussed unless your physician suggests otherwise.

That said, treatment and prevention of osteoporosis is directed at stimulating or assisting the friendly osteoblasts to get on with their work of producing bone—and discouraging those nasty little osteoclasts from taking bone away from us. To do this, we have to give the osteoblasts the appropriate tools, the most important of which (in addition to calcium and vitamin D) are exercise, bone-sparing medications, and other precautionary measures.

While accelerated bone loss is associated with diets deficient in calcium or vitamin D and disorders that impair the absorption, knowledge of other demineralizing influences can enable us to employ some of these precautionary measures. For example: The excessive ingestion of vitamin A and cigarette smoking can increase the risk of bone loss and osteoporosis. Recent research also suggests that women who drink more than three cups of coffee a day may further decrease their bone density. People who are immobilized due to illness and those who have a sedentary lifestyle (as in the case of couch potatoes) are also subject to a more pronounced loss of bone.

Resistance training and osteoporosis

Resistance training and other forms of exercise that enhance osteoblastic activity can be extremely important in fighting osteoporosis. In one study, the bone density of the femoral neck, where so many fractures occur, was increased by 3.8 percent after just 16 weeks of resistance training. In another study that involved postmenopausal women from 50 to 70 years old, the bone mineral density of the lumbar spine was increased by 6.3 percent after one year of training. During this same period of time, the control group that was *not* involved in the training program experienced a 3.7 percent loss of bone mineral density. This amounted to an actual difference of 10 percent between those who were in training and those who did not train. Other studies have shown similar results, even in women who are not taking estrogen. Because strong muscles are associated with strong bones, strengthening our muscles will, in turn, strengthen our bones.Walking, jogging, vibration training, and a host of other exercises that we'll discuss later can strengthen your muscles and your bones—so let's get ready.

The important thing to remember is that prevention is better than cure. Retarding the progress of—or even preventing—osteoporosis with some of the measures we've discussed is far easier and more effective than treating advanced osteoporosis after it has become established.

Bone-sparing medications

In established osteoporosis, a hormone called *calcitonin* can be taken by nasal spray along with calcium supplements. This hormone can increase bone density and prevent fractures. An even more effective group of medicines known as the *biphosphonates* (Didronel, Fosamax, etc.) have met with great success. When taken with calcium and vitamin D, these drugs can increase bone density and bone strength. They work by decreasing the activity of the osteoclasts (the little buggers that take bone away), and they've been shown to decrease fractures of the wrist and hip. So you see, once again, the objectives of treatment are to enhance the activity of our friendly osteoblasts and to decrease the activity of those villainous osteoclasts.

More recently, a medication called Evista (raloxifene) has shown very promising results in treating osteoporosis. Its effects are similar to estrogen for producing bone and preventing bone loss. But its effects are *anti-estrogen* on breast and uterine tissue. So as it improves bone mineral density, it may also protect against breast cancer. As an important word of caution, these drugs are prescription medications. They all have significant side effects and should only be taken under careful medical supervision.

There's yet another interesting development on the horizon. Observational studies suggest that a class of medication called *statins* (used to treat high cholesterol) may also have a beneficial effect on bone density. Patients taking this type of medication appear to have a much lower incidence of fractures and greater degree of bone mineral density. So it may be that statins inhibit the action of osteoclasts. While there is much research yet to be done on this subject, I am hopeful that the observational findings of these preliminary reports are documented by more targeted studies. Since statins have comparatively few side effects, they—or some pharmacological modification of them—could turn out to be a boon to the treatment and the prevention of osteoporosis in the future.

OSTEOARTHRITIS

Understandably, some people confuse *osteoporosis* and *osteoarthritis*. After all, the first five letters of both words are the same—and both maladies frequent the same age group. Osteoarthritis, commonly referred to as degenerative arthritis, usually involves the fingers, knees, hips, shoulders, and spine. It is primarily a disorder of the joints—not the bones—and shares no relationship to osteoporosis. With the wear and tear of time, the cartilage that cushions our joints becomes roughened and pitted and begins to degenerate. The decrease in the cushioning of the joints results in a grating of the bones that make up the involved joint. This added stress and irritation of the joint's bony surfaces stimulates an overgrowth of bone spurs and *osteophytes*, fragments of bone often referred to as "joint mice." (As an interesting side note, this disease is not limited to human beings. It would appear that osteoarthritis actually evolved along with the vertebrate skeleton, because it has also been found in prehistoric dinosaurs, whales, fish, and birds.)

Symptoms can begin as early as the third decade and are common by the age of 40. By the age of 70, almost everybody has developed some osteoarthritis. The term "degenerative arthritis" serves to clearly differentiate it from inflammatory diseases of the joints such as *rheumatoid arthritis*—the other disorder with which it is often confused. To be clear, osteoarthritis bears no relationship to rheumatoid arthritis or similar inflammatory joint diseases.

Symptoms

While osteoarthritis is usually a slowly progressive disorder, it can stop or even reverse. The onset of pain is gradual. At first, morning stiffness usually decreases after 15 to 20 minutes of activity. Limitation of motion, joint swelling, increasing pain on motion, and joint tenderness can become more apparent as the condition progresses.

Treatment

PHYSICAL THERAPY

Various forms of physical therapy (exercise, cold packs, hot packs, massage, acupuncture, etc.) are the mainstay of treatment and have proven to be successful in most cases. Stretching exercises that preserve the range of motion and resistance exercises that help to strengthen the muscles and stabilize the joint are very effective. Back, wrist, or knee supports can also be beneficial.

While drug therapy is the least important aspect of treatment, pain can often be alleviated with analgesics. Tylenol, aspirin, or nonsteroidal anti-inflammatory drugs, commonly referred to as NSAIDs or COX-1 inhibitors (Motrin, Naprosyn, etc.), may be used—but their continued use may have adverse effects. NSAIDs can cause kidney damage, and both aspirin and NSAIDs may irritate your gastrointestinal tract and cause ulcers and bleeding. A newer variety of NSAIDs called COX-2 inhibitors are less likely to cause gastrointestinal irritation, but some have been linked to an increase in heart attacks and strokes.

Be cautious, because all of these drugs can have serious side effects. Check with your doctor before using them on a continuous basis. And try to stay away from strong pain relievers such as narcotics or narcotic-like drugs. Habituation, reliance, and addiction are easy to come by—but very hard to leave behind.

On a relatively different note, a member of the tetracycline group of antibiotics, known as *doxycycline*, seems to slow or even prevent the progression of osteoarthritis. It's believed to work by blocking some of the enzymes that break down cartilage. Extensive research is in progress to determine the effectiveness of this antibiotic, but the jury is still out.

CHONDROITIN AND GLUCOSAMINE

Several reports suggest that the combination of chondroitin sulfate and glucosamine can be helpful in osteoarthritis. Chondroitin sulfate is an important ingredient in the cartilage and connective tissue of all animals. Glucosamine serves as a building block for many of the constituents that make up the joints and joint fluids. About 25 percent of people with early joint disease seem to feel better taking these agents. The combination tablet can be purchased in almost any pharmacy without a prescription. Since I don't know of any serious toxicity associated with these ingredients, I think they're worth a try.

INJECTIONS

The injection of cortisone drugs directly into the joint may be helpful when swelling or other signs of inflammation are present. Generally, these drugs are used intermittently and as infrequently as possible.

On a different note, a substance called *hyaluronic acid,* which is a normal constituent of joint fluid, has proven very helpful. In a large number of patients, intra-articular injections of commercial preparations of hyaluronic acid (Hyalgan, Artz, Synvisc) have resulted in a measurable and surprisingly sustained improvement.

ALTERNATIVE THERAPY

While it may not alter the course of the disease, acupuncture has helped many patients by relieving the pain secondary to osteoarthritis. In this role, it can serve as a valuable adjunct to a good physiotherapy program. Other alternative therapies are questionable, however. An example: The claim made by many naturopaths that specific diets, herbs, and vitamin supplements can successfully treat osteoarthritis is without any scientific proof, so I can't recommend it. If you're going to use this kind of therapy, please check with your doctor to make sure he or she knows what you're taking and what you're doing.

WEIGHT REDUCTION

It is well-known that osteoarthritis can be more severe in obese people. Why? Because of the added pressure on joints. A nutritious, low-calorie diet can help to reduce stress on weight-bearing joints, thereby decreasing pain and even slowing down the progress of the disease.

SURGERY

In the event that conservative therapy fails, osteoarthritis can progress with increasing pain, severe limitation of motion, and a mounting compromise of one's ability to ambulate. At this point surgery can be of enormous value in restoring quality of life. A minimally invasive procedure known as *arthroscopy* involves the insertion of a special scope into the joint space to remove fragments of cartilage and other debris. While the downtime is considerably less than with open surgical procedures, some recent studies have questioned its effectiveness.

In more advanced cases, an *arthroplasty* can be performed. This open surgery to repair the joint can frequently produce wonderful long-term improvement. In even more advanced osteoarthritis, partial or even total joint replacement may be preferable. In more than 90 percent of cases, complete replacement of knee joints, hip joints, and shoulder joints have been successful. Before undergoing any of these procedures, however—and particularly before becoming the bionic man or woman—be sure to consult with a good rheumatologist. If it's determined that you need surgery, make sure you have an orthopedic surgeon who is experienced in these procedures.

LOOKING BACK, LOOKING FORWARD

CHAPTER 9 REVIEW ...

◆ Hormone replacement therapy (HRT) has real dangers that must be carefully considered by both the doctor and the patient.

◆ A supplementary combination of calcium and vitamin D—along with a regular exercise program—can prevent bone loss due to osteoporosis.

◆ Cigarette smoking, excessive intake of vitamin A or coffee, and a sedentary lifestyle increase the risk of osteoporosis.

◆ Various forms of physical therapy are the mainstay treatments for osteoarthritis.

CHAPTER 10 PREVIEW ...

◆ What causes wrinkles and age spots? What's the best way to prevent further skin damage— or to repair damage already done?

◆ Are there any serious side effects from chemical peels, lasers, or injections?

◆ Is sun exposure really as dangerous as some people say?

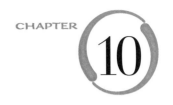

SKIN: SPOTS, DOTS, AND AGING

*Age imprints more wrinkles in the
mind than it does on the face.*
—Michel de Montaigne

*I'm tired of all this nonsense about beauty
being only skin-deep. That's deep enough.
What do you want, an adorable pancreas?*
—Jean Kerr

THE SKIN

Before discussing wrinkle remedies, let's talk a little about our aging skin in general. Most of the effects of aging on the skin are attributable more to sun exposure than to actual aging. The more appropriate term for these changes is probably *photo-aging*. The effects include a variety of colored spots, roughening of the skin surface, and sagging or wrinkling of the skin due to a loss of elasticity.

Many of the discolored, rough spots we get are called *keratoses*—unkindly referred to as "senile keratoses" because they progressively appear on our skin as we age. Most of these are benign lesions that are of no real consequence beyond their cosmetic appearance. It is essential, however, that they be differentiated from more serious skin lesions such as skin cancer or another type of keratoses called *actinic keratoses*. Some dermatologists consider this type of keratoses to be precancerous or actually a form of cancer itself.

Skin cancer

Skin cancer is very common. That's why it is very, very important to recognize the serious effects of sun exposure. While there are many different types of skin cancer, some are much more dangerous than others. Three types are clearly related to sun exposure. *Basal cell carcinoma* is a locally invasive cancer that spreads only in very rare instances and can almost always be treated effectively by your general practitioner or by a dermatologist. Another type, *squamous cell carcinoma,* can spread if not detected and treated early. Cure rates are also very good for this type of cancer. The third type, called a *melanoma,* is really dangerous. A melanoma usually appears as a nevus, or pigmented spot or mole. If not treated early, it can spread to distant parts of the body—and it can be fatal. Recent advances in gene therapy (derived from our understanding of the human genome), however, have shown promising results in about one-third of patients. The upshot is that hope is on the way. *The important thing to remember is this: If a spot on your skin changes in size, changes in color, begins to itch, or concerns you in any other way, please have your doctor take a look at it.* Early diagnosis and treatment are the keys to cure.

Sunscreen

Considering the risks, why would you want to be a sun-bather? Sure, a little bit of sun can be a good way to get vitamin D—but bathing in the sun to get a deep tan or going to tanning parlors for cosmetic reasons is irrational. Many of us baked on the beach when we were kids, and today's young people are still out there on the beach, broiling in the sun. *This is downright dangerous.* It increases the chance of getting skin cancer, wrinkles, crows feet, keratoses, and God knows what else. If any of you are still doing this, please stop it! And if you know people, young or old, who are still doing it—tell them to stop it!

What can we do if our work or favorite activities, such as golf or tennis, take us out into the sun? *A simple answer is to wear protective clothing and a brimmed hat to shield your face.* Also cover all the exposed surfaces of your skin with a good sunscreening cream or lotion.

The ultraviolet (UV) rays that damage your skin are primarily of two types: UV-A rays and UV-B rays. It's the UV-B rays that cause sunburn. The UV-A rays penetrate through the upper layers of the skin and cause the deeper damage responsible for photo-aging. So it's important that the sunscreen you choose provides good protection against both UV-A and UV-B rays. If you're not sure, check with your doctor or pharmacist.

Wear sunscreen every day. Your skin gets exposed even on cloudy days or while you're riding in your car (windows screen out some of the rays, but not all of them). Regular use of a good protective lotion can do more than prevent further photo-aging and decrease your chances of getting skin cancer. It might actually reverse some of the damage your skin has already suffered.

Treating wrinkles

What's the best line of defense against developing "old skin" while treating some of the changes that occur? You guessed right: *It's protection from the rays of the sun.* In terms of actually *treating* wrinkles, I don't know if expensive facial massages or fancy mudpacks from the caves of Shangri La can actually make a difference. Many people try such things in an effort to look better. I have no problem with that. After all, that's why we comb our hair. And realistically, there's some merit in this: For many people, concern for their appearance has a positive effect on their level of self-confidence and self-esteem. That's reason enough to touch on this subject.

PEELS, LASERS, AND INJECTIONS

Chemical peels using glycolic acid and the use of some of the newer laser, radio-frequency, and heat treatments can be very effective in erasing minor spots, wrinkles, and even reducing furrows. The reduction in wrinkles seems to work by inducing the production of collagen. Some such treatments can even reduce cellulite and fat deposits in certain parts of the body. While the results are less pronounced than a surgical facelift or surgical liposuction, they are considerably less expensive and have little or no downtime. Some treatments require mild sedation and topical anesthetics and are associated with some swelling and discomfort. This can be bothersome, but it usually disappears in a few days. In using this technology, many dermatologists indicate that maximum effectiveness can be achieved using the *ReFirme* device for facial work and the

VelaSmooth machine for body contouring. Their preference for these particular devices is based on the fact that no sedation or anesthetic is required and neither appears to be associated with significant discomfort or downtime.

Furrows can also be reduced and some wrinkles even erased by injecting *collagen* preparations or fillers such as Restyiane, Juvéderm, etc., directly into and around the wrinkle or injecting Botox into selected facial muscles. A point of interest: Botox is the pharmaceutical preparation of the food poison that causes botulism. This rare disease can cause fatal paralysis of muscles when food contaminated by the bacteria known as *Clostridium botulinum* is eaten.

Botox presents no such risk. The pharmaceutical preparation for this popular wrinkle treatment is quite safe in experienced hands. When the Botox is injected into selected facial muscles, the subsequent relaxation of the muscles allows many furrows and wrinkles to decrease or even disappear. It should be noted, however, that the effects of filler injections into wrinkles or Botox injections into facial muscles are not permanent; the procedure may have to be repeated in several months.

ANTIWRINKLE CREAMS

Certain acids such as lactic acid, citric acid, or AHAs (alpha-hydroxy acids) have been shown to reduce the wrinkling and the thinning of skin that accompanies aging. They appear to work quite well in many people. So far, however, the only magic in a tube is Retin-A cream. When used daily for several months it has been effective in reducing small wrinkles and pigmentations and may also reverse the growth of the precancerous skin condition called actinic keratoses. The longer this cream is used, the greater the benefit. Retin-A concentrations of 0.05 percent are more effective than concentrations of 0.02 percent but are more likely to be associated with swelling and redness. However, with continued use, this side effect usually disappears over a period of three to four months.

PLASTIC SURGERY

Redundant skin around your neck (the so-called "turkey neck"), deep wrinkles or furrows, sagging jowls, and sagging eyelids cannot be cured by any antiwrinkle creams or lotions. The only effective way to alter these conditions is with cosmetic surgery—often called reconstructive or plastic surgery. It should be noted that significant advances have been made in cosmetic surgical techniques; the discomfort and the recovery time are much less than they used to be, and the results can be very gratifying.

A word to the wise: If you are contemplating any of these procedures, be absolutely certain that the therapist you've selected has good credentials and lots of experience in this type of work. Although infrequent, these treatments are not without side effects and complications. A fair warning: Too much bargain hunting and a failure to thoroughly investigate could result in undesirable consequences.

LOOKING BACK, LOOKING FORWARD

CHAPTER 10 REVIEW ◆ ◆ ◆

◆ Any spot on the skin that itches or changes in size or color should be examined by a doctor.

◆ Skin creams containing Retin-A, lactic acid, citric acid, or AHAs may reduce age-related wrinkling and thinning of the skin.

◆ Daily use of a sunscreen lotion or cream can prevent skin cancer and reduce the effects of aging.

◆ Cosmetic procedures such as chemical peels and filler injections can decrease wrinkles and serve as an important adjunct to a person's self-esteem and sense of wellbeing.

CHAPTER 11 PREVIEW ◆ ◆ ◆

◆ Is it possible to significantly develop muscle strength without looking like a bodybuilder?

◆ How is aerobic exercise different from anaerobic exercise? Is one kind better than the other?

◆ What are the relative advantages of high- and low-impact exercise routines?

◆ Why is it wise to check with your doctor before undertaking an exercise program? What pre-existing medical conditions can make some exercises dangerous?

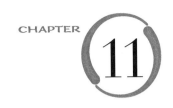

ABOUT EXERCISE

*Those who do not find time for exercise
will have to find time for illness.*

–The Earl of Derby

I have two doctors—my left leg and my right.

–Anonymous

Exercise is not an option—it's an absolute imperative. We *must* maintain or improve our strength, our endurance, our balance, and our flexibility. Why? *Talk about a giant payoff!* Exercise may or may not enable you to live longer, but it will surely enable you to live better. It's likely to add years to your life, and it's absolutely certain to add life to your years. At any age, exercise is a major factor in compressing morbidity (suffering fewer illnesses and more rapidly recovering from illness). *Of all of the healthful things you can do, regular exercise is probably the one that's most important.*

As an example: Who doesn't know the terrible health consequences of cigarette smoking? Yet some studies have shown that men who smoke cigarettes—but also exercise regularly—are better off than nonsmokers who don't exercise. Clearly, cigarette smoking is a dreadful addiction. (I can attest to that on a personal level.) Because it is associated with deadly diseases, tobacco is a major societal health hazard. Anyone who smokes should make every effort to stop. Those who fail should try and try again; if they stick to it, they'll succeed. Having said that, the suggestion that fitness appears to have an even greater effect on improving longevity and decreasing morbidity further underscores the value of regular exercise. You can get stronger and have more vigor, more vitality, and greater mental clarity.

IT'S NOT TOO LATE TO START

No matter how old you are or how much damage your body may already have suffered, it's never too late. "Couch potatoes" who don't begin to exercise until their 40s or even their 70s can get in better shape than the high school and college jocks they knew who gave up exercising. While it's true that the early bird catches the worm—it's also true that the second mouse gets the cheese. *This is your chance—your chance to get the cheese.* Exercise can make a spectacular improvement in your conditioning and the way you feel and look. You will thank your Maker over and over again for the enormous resources preserved in your body—resources that you can call upon at almost any age—that will improve your strength and fitness in an amazingly short period of time. You can definitely—d-e-f-i-n-i-t-e-l-y—be Nifty after Fifty. Friends and family will be infected by the change in your appearance, the spring in your step, and your renewed energy. Perhaps it will encourage them to emulate you by getting started on an exercise program themselves.

If you're young, the best time to start is now. Likewise, if you're in your sixties or in your nineties, the best time to start is now. Many of us have children who are anywhere from 20 to 60 years old. We've taught them morals and table manners. We taught them not to interrupt people, to brush their teeth, and to chew with their mouths closed. We taught them to look both ways before crossing the street. And we didn't teach these things just by *talking*. We taught them by *example*. Now we can teach them something equally important—far more important to their long-term wellbeing and their survival. We can teach them the value of regular exercise, but *you must do so by example.*

ENDORPHINS

Most of us regular exercisers don't really like to exercise. We only think we like to exercise because we love the way it makes us feel. That's partly because of *endorphins* (opioid peptides). Endorphins are mostly produced in our pituitary gland, but also in some parts of the brain. That's why scientists believe they also play an important role in emotions, memory, and learning. (They're not really related to opium or morphine, by the way, but they act at the same receptor sites in our body.)

Our bodies seem to produce more of these natural substances when we exercise. Scientists think it's the release of endorphins that makes us feel so good when we work out. Endorphins are almost addicting. That's probably one of the reasons people who regularly exercise don't feel as well if they skip too many workouts. They miss the invigorated feeling, the wonderful *high,* and the antidepressant effect of their own natural endorphins. People who get into it and keep going for 8 to 16 weeks love the way it makes them feel—so they tend to keep at it.

EXERCISE BENEFITS ALL BODY SYSTEMS

Physical exercise affects more than just muscles and bones. Remember that, as the brain ages, there's a decrease in the formation of both dendrites and synapses (the branching and connecting of our brain and nerve cells). Did you know it was once believed that after maturity, the brain had no ability to grow? Now we know differently. Now we know that physical and mental exercise can stimulate the production of a substance called *brain growth factor* and improve brain function at almost any age.

In addition to increasing blood flow to the brain, physical exercise turns on that amazing computer between our ears and clicks on all the right symbols! Every time your muscles contract, they release a substance called IGF-1. This protein substance enters the bloodstream and travels to the brain, where it stimulates the production of another substance called brain-derived neurotrophic factor (BDNF). This substance stimulates the growth and branching of the brain cells and multiplies the number of synapses or connections between them. Without a doubt, physical exercise—working out regularly—has a very positive effect on brain function, particularly as we age. It may not make you smarter, but it will certainly improve your brain function so that you can become smarter if you try.

All of the above goes to show that physical exercise can have a remarkably positive effect on many different body systems. While improving our muscle and bone strength and balance, exercise also has the marvelous effect of elevating our good cholesterol and decreasing our bad cholesterol. It improves our cardiac function and our lung or pulmonary function—one of the most important determinants in increasing longevity and decreasing morbidity. What's more, strength and endurance training actually improves the functioning of our gastrointestinal tract and our metabolism.

Strength training, in particular, increases your muscle mass, which in turn increases your metabolic rate. This enables you to burn more calories and fat even at rest—because *resting muscle burns more calories than resting fat.* Studies have also shown increased insulin sensitivity and improved glucose tolerance in people on strength training programs. So if you suffer from diabetes, do yourself a favor and seriously consider strength training. It can improve your sugar metabolism and reduce your insulin requirements.

STRENGTH TRAINING PREVENTS PROBLEMS

Let's talk a little about the importance of strengthening muscles. Between the ages of 40 and 70 most men and women will lose about 30 percent to 50 percent of their strength. That's an average of 1 percent to 1.5 percent each year.

What a depressing fact! *But the loss is not irreversible*—and that's really exciting. This progressive loss of strength is associated with diminished muscle mass, a condition called *sarcopenia.* The development of sarcopenia is accelerated by the inactivity that too often accompanies aging—which, of course, can be even further accelerated by chronic disease. As chronic problems such as arthritis, emphysema, diabetes, and heart disease discourage activity, the result is further worsening of sarcopenia.

Loss of muscle strength leads to a decrease in endurance and balance. Ultimately, this strength-endurance-balance deficit impairs functionality and increases falls. Approximately one out of every three seniors will experience a fall each year. As we age, falls and fractures become one of the leading causes of death— and above the age of 85, falls are the *major* cause. Remember that weak muscles are also associated with weak bones (osteoporosis). Osteoporosis is associated with a greater frequency of fractures, more severe fractures, and the poor healing of fractures. Even in elderly people, strength training can improve bone density, muscle strength, and balance. The bottom line: *Strength training has the potential to reduce the likelihood of falls and fractures and the grief that accompanies them.*

I'm not suggesting that anyone who exercises can become an Arnold Schwarzenegger; that's not going to happen. And women aren't going to become muscular or masculinized Amazons, either—not unless they set out to get that effect. Even if it's more likely that you can prevent osteoporosis if you start early, the benefits for the elderly are enormous as well. Studies show that even if you're between the ages of 80 and 90 you can increase your leg strength by more than 100 percent in just 8 to 16 weeks of supervised training. In the participants of one study, walking speed increased by 28 percent and stair-climbing ability increased by 12 percent or more. *Some of these subjects actually threw away their walkers and canes.* That's what I call a good example of the second mouse grabbing the cheese! Not only did their strength improve, but their balance also improved—probably because greater muscle strength was associated with greater joint stability.

Other studies have shown equally beneficial effects on bone density. As mentioned earlier, the bone density of the neck of the femur (thigh bone) can be increased by 3.8 percent in just 16 weeks of strength training. In a group of postmenopausal women, the bone density of the lower back (the lumbar spine) was increased by 6.3 percent after just one year of strength training. It should also be noted that the control group of women in this study (women who did not participate in strength training) *lost* 3.7 percent of their bone density during this same period of time. *In only a year, that's a total difference of 10 percent in bone density between the women on a strength-training program and the inactive group.* Upper-body strength training will also improve bone density. Why is this so important? *Remember that most fractures in older men and women occur in the hips, wrists, arms, shoulders, and lower spine.*

We can't afford *not* to find the time for regular exercise! The average adult in this country spends some three to four hours a day watching TV or surfing the Internet. Ouch! Think about the Surgeon General's warning label on cigarettes. Well, I think the Surgeon General should also put a warning on the TV screen that says, "Watching television, combined with failure to exercise on a regular basis, can accelerate obesity, heart disease, lung disease, diabetes, dementia, osteoporosis, falls, fractures, and death."

OTHER TYPES OF EXERCISE

A healthy heart and healthy lungs are crucial to longevity and your ongoing quality of life. You can further pave the path to heart health through endurance training—also called aerobic or cardiopulmonary training. The fact is that about 40 percent of us will probably die from some type of cardiovascular disease. *Endurance training might cut that risk in half.*

Yoga, brisk walking, jogging, stair-stepping, and cycling exercises are good examples. For most of these, all you need is a good pair of shoes. Stretching exercises that improve flexibility, especially when augmented by balance exercises, will reduce the incidence of injuries and falls. Working together, strength training, endurance training, stretching, and balance training are an excellent method of achieving a greater level of fitness.

About 20 percent of all of us will be classified as "frail" when we get older. Even if we don't become frail, we're going to be a lot weaker with the passing years. (It should be noted that frailty can descend upon any of us quite suddenly, as a result of illness or an accident.) Those of us who do become frail will account for 40 percent to 50 percent of health-care expenditures. Whether we suffer from heart disease, lung disease, arthritis, liver disease, kidney disease, neurological disease, diabetes, or whatever—there's a common denominator to that frailty. It's *muscle weakness!* It's sarcopenia.

Just think about the ways a person's primary disease process can be gravely aggravated by muscle weakness. Suppose you fall. Even if you don't sustain a fracture, you may not have the strength to get up. Some of us will suddenly find ourselves unable to rise from a chair or the toilet seat! That sets up the need for assisted living—and the loss of our independence.

Having just discussed some of the relevant studies, we now know that strength training can reverse a lot of this muscle weakness. Not only will it *prevent* catastrophes, strength training will help us *survive* a catastrophe! We, all of us, *have to do it.* I promise that once you get started, you'll love it, and you'll never want to stop.

Those of us who are in pretty good shape can start an exercise program that combines strength training, stretching exercises, endurance training, and balance exercises at the same time. But many of us won't be able to do this. We can't effectively perform balance and endurance exercises because of a lack of strength. In this case, improving our strength is the first order of business. Stronger muscles will equip us to perform balance and endurance exercises at a later time.

Strength training, however, can and should be combined with stretching exercises to improve flexibility. Both have a highly beneficial effect on balance. With the addition of special balance exercises, the results can be spectacular. It goes without saying that weak leg muscles can't effectively perform aerobic exercises such as jogging, stair-climbing, or even brisk walking. Lower-body strength training is necessary to prepare the leg muscles for these exercises and further improvement.

AEROBIC AND ANAEROBIC EXERCISE

It's really important to understand that strength training and cardiopulmonary training should be viewed as complementary rather than mutually exclusive. Both objectives can be achieved. A strength-training program, for example, can be configured to also give you a good cardiopulmonary workout. Alternatively, strength and aerobic workouts can be done on alternate days.

MUSCLE PHYSIOLOGY

Have I convinced you yet of the marvelous effects of cardiopulmonary training and resistance training? Perhaps it will help if I explain a little muscle physiology—about how the muscle cell breathes and the chemical process through which energy is produced and utilized by the muscle cell. Do you remember our prior discussion about carbohydrate metabolism? I explained how sugars and starches are converted to a substance called glycogen, and how the glycogen stored in our muscles serves as a bank of stored energy.

What happens when we contract a muscle? One of the first steps in the liberation of energy for muscle contraction is the breakdown of the glycogen stored in our muscle fibers. This occurs through a series of very complex chemical reactions that involve enzymes and catalysts. As we exercise our muscles, they utilize energy and produce a chemical called *lactic acid* or *lactate*. Muscle lactate is, so to speak, the metabolic "end product" of the exercising muscle.

As we inhale, oxygen enters our lungs and is carried by our blood throughout our body. What happens when the oxygen gets to our muscles? It clears the lactate. So if there is an adequate amount of oxygen and a lesser amount of lactate, the lactate won't accumulate. What I'm describing is *aerobic muscle contraction* (muscle contraction in the presence of oxygen). If exercise is rapid or vigorous and the oxygen supply is inadequate to keep up with the formation of lactate, lactate accumulates in the muscle. Muscle contraction in the absence of sufficient oxygen is what is meant by *anaerobic muscle contraction*.

Not surprisingly, our muscles use oxygen at an increased rate when we exercise. The harder and longer we exercise, the harder we breathe in an effort to get more oxygen to our muscles—to clear the lactate.

If the exercising muscle produces lactate faster than oxygen can be supplied, a so-called "oxygen debt" is created in the muscle—and lactate accumulates. The muscle may feel tired or tight due to an accumulation of lactate. Continued exercise of the muscle in this state (anaerobic exercise) unleashes a cascade of physiologic events that stimulate muscle growth and strength, as happens in resistance training.

Resting the muscle reduces the rate of lactate formation, and deep breathing brings more oxygen to the muscle, helping to clear the lactate and to decrease the fatigue. That's the recovery phase of the muscle—the payback of the *oxygen debt.*

Because of this fantastic mechanism, our muscles are able to contract and perform work even in the absence of sufficient oxygen (unlike the motor-driven engines we've invented). But our muscles do depend on a continuous and contemporaneous supply of oxygen. As an example: The maximum amount of oxygen that can be exchanged by us mortals is about four liters a minute. But an athlete who sprints 100 yards in 11 seconds may use six liters of oxygen in that brief moment in time. After the sprint, the athlete pants and breathes deeply, repaying the oxygen debt over the next several minutes.

Theoretically, if oxygen is brought to the exercising muscles and clears the lactate at the same rate that the muscle produces it, no lactate is accumulated and there is no oxygen debt. This "pay as you go" mechanism is aerobic exercise—exercise with oxygen. Carefully paced exercises that use the larger muscles of the body, such as the leg muscles, are best employed for such exercises. Some good examples are treadmill exercises, brisk walking, jogging, cycling, and stair-stepping—among many others. But if any of these exercises are performed too fast or too long, an anaerobic phase will be entered; lactate accumulation, oxygen debt, and muscle fatigue will develop.

If you're doing an aerobic or cardiopulmonary workout, there's no point in entering into an anaerobic phase. In fact, you want to forestall it. While there's no foolproof way of telling when this is happening, a simple rule of thumb is this: While you're exercising, you should have sufficient breath to carry on a normal conversation with someone standing next to you. If you can't do that, the chances are you are entering an anaerobic phase of exercise. To correct that, you should slow down—and if that doesn't seem to work, you should stop. When you're able to resume that imaginary conversation, go ahead and resume the exercise at a slower pace.

EXERCISE AND CALORIC EXPENDITURE

You can probably burn more calories in a 30-minute cardiopulmonary workout than you can in an hour or more of strength training. But that's not the whole story. Remember that muscles burn more calories at rest, and larger muscles burn even more calories at rest. By increasing your strength and the muscle mass of your body through strength training, you will actually burn *more* calories at rest. Why? Your RMR will increase.

EXERCISE AND MUSCLE SIZE

Some people are afraid to get into strength training because of the misconception that they will get to look like a bodybuilder with big bulging muscles. Although I think a well-muscled body is good-looking, building big muscles takes a lot more gym time than what we're talking about. Serious bodybuilders commonly spend three to six hours a day in the gym—and that's five to six days a week! I'm suggesting a strength-training program that takes about 30 minutes two to four times a week. There's just no comparison. Studies done on women have repeatedly shown that using strength training to increase the muscle mass of their thighs did not increase the actual *size* of their thighs. In fact, their thighs either got smaller or stayed the same size, but were better toned—more firm. Do you understand what happened? As muscle mass increased, the fat mass decreased. Here's a little rap ditty that sums it all up. It goes like this:

> *On a pound of fat, let me make my case.*
> *A pound of muscle takes less space.*
> *A pound of muscle, you soon will learn,*
> *Hastens the pace of the fat you burn.*
> *So listen up, cat, and hear my chat.*
> *A pound of muscle is where it's at.*
> *A pound of fat is a pound of fat.*
> *A pound of fat is only that.*

HIGH- AND LOW-IMPACT EXERCISES

Jogging and running are great cardiopulmonary exercises, but they're considered high-impact exercise—which means they might be responsible for causing joint damage. While there is some merit to these concerns, there's also some value to impact. Exercise associated with impact helps to stimulate those wonderful little osteoblasts (cells that produce healthy bone). We have already discussed how strength-training exercises increase bone density.

But we're not so sure about low-impact exercise. Low-impact exercises such as swimming, brisk walking, cycling, and stair-stepping are excellent in terms of a cardiopulmonary workout and in reducing joint stress. They may, however, have a lesser effect on preventing osteoporosis. I often recommend that people who rely on low-impact exercises for their total workout consider jogging in place for 60 seconds a day. If you have a knee or a back problem—or any kind of joint problems—you should check with your doctor. He or she should help you decide what exercises are safe for you.

WHO SHOULD EXERCISE? ARE THERE ANY PRECAUTIONS?

Thomas Jefferson said, "Exercise and recreation . . . are as necessary as reading. I will rather say more necessary, because health is worth more than learning." This statement was made about 200 years ago. I'm not sure about the value of making such a comparison, but it emphasizes the enormous respect the president, who was a science scholar, had for exercise.

There are very few exceptions to the rule that almost everyone should be involved in regular exercise—regardless of their age or ailments. The Surgeon General has reported that failure to exercise, no matter how old you are, might be one of our greatest health hazards. What about those of you who have chronic disorders such as heart disease, lung disease, and arthritis? Exercise can be of benefit to you as well, but it should be avoided during flare-ups of your illness or what doctors call *exacerbations.* You can resume your exercise program when you and your doctor believe your flare-up has subsided.

Stability is the important thing for those of us with a chronic condition. Is the condition stable or not? If the condition is stable, you can start or resume an exercise program. If you have a chronic disease, by the way, you want to make it your business to know all about it—you have to be educated. It's important to know the specific dangers and the signs that suggest that a flare-up is starting. You and your doctor have to discuss these things until you understand them thoroughly. If a situation develops and you're in doubt as to its importance, it's best to check with your doctor. He or she may want you to come in for a checkup before you start or resume your exercise program.

MILD, MODERATE, AND VIGOROUS EXERCISE

Mild to moderate exercise can benefit almost anyone; vigorous exercise will benefit most of us even more! Some studies show that people who indulge in mild to moderate activity seem to age as well as those who indulge in more vigorous exercise. These are observational studies that looked at populations who were involved in walking clubs, gardening clubs, and similar endeavors—all wonderful activities.

But you and I are individuals; each and every one of us is. As such, the best condition you are in, *as an individual*, the better off you will be. Of course this can be carried to an extreme. I'm talking about *fitness for health*—not *fitness for fitness*. For example, the training program of a professional boxer is *fitness for fitness* training. A boxer training for a championship fight wants to be in better condition than his opponent in the last round of the fight. While we can appreciate the merit of his endeavor, there's no evidence that his extreme level of fitness provides him with any additional health benefits.

Generally speaking, a reasonable set of guidelines is as follows: Exercise that makes you sweat a lot or makes you short of breath is *vigorous exercise*. Exercise that produces a mild sweat or leaves you slightly winded is *moderate exercise*. Exercise that does neither is *mild exercise*. Now we should all be aware that mild exercise for one person may be vigorous exercise for another. Also, some of us tend to sweat much more easily than others. So the application of these guidelines has to be individualized and judged by your own experience.

One thing is clear. It's important to start gradually and to avoid hurting yourself by overactivity. Any good exercise program is likely to be associated with some mild muscular discomfort, but rushing into vigorous exercise can cause pain and actual injury. This can put you on the sidelines and cancel out the progress you've made. Even worse, it can create negative psychological feedback that can cause you to avoid exercise altogether. So let's agree to approach exercise *gradually*—and gradually build on the gain we achieve.

CAUTION: WHEN *NOT* TO EXERCISE!

It must be said that in a small subset of people, strength training could be hazardous; an even smaller subset should avoid any type of vigorous exertion. Some pertinent examples are individuals with *uncontrolled high blood pressure, certain uncontrolled heart arrythmias, damaged heart valves, aortic aneurysms, unstable angina, recent or untreated congestive heart failure (CHF), and, as previously stated, people currently suffering a flare-up of a chronic condition.* For example: If you have rheumatoid arthritis and develop a red-hot or inflamed joint, you shouldn't be exercising at all until the flare-up has subsided.

Here are some further notes on a few of the conditions already mentioned.

Aortic aneurysms: The aorta is the main artery going out from the heart, as shown in this illustration. It travels down the chest, through the diaphragm and into the abdomen, giving off branches that supply blood to all parts of the body. Sometimes a weakening in the wall of this major blood vessel occurs,

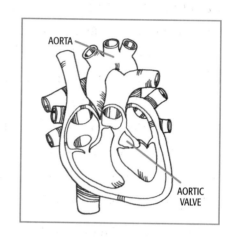

causing a "ballooning out" or bubble formation. In this circumstance, exertion could cause a rupture or break that could be fatal—as it was for the world-renowned scientist, Albert Einstein. Even in this case, however, someone who has a very small aneurysm, or one that has been surgically repaired, can consult a doctor who could prescribe certain exercises that would be safe.

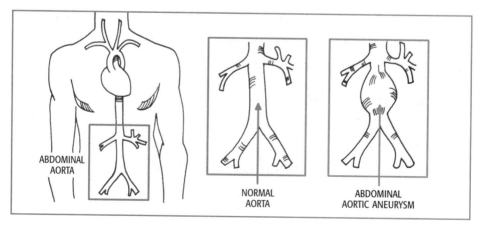

Heart valve damage: The heart has four valves, as shown in the illustration. Certain diseases such as rheumatic fever can damage these valves. Sometimes the damage is of such a magnitude that it interferes with the flow of blood into or out of the heart. The impediment to blood flow varies with the severity of the damage. If you have such a condition, you should consult your physician before taking on any exercise program.

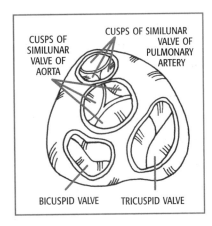

The same can be said about *coronary artery disease*, which can be associated with angina pectoris (usually characterized by chest pain on exertion). In mild cases, limited exercise often improves exertional tolerance. But if the angina recurs more frequently or more severely or with less exertion than previously experienced, it should be checked. As I'm sure you can appreciate, this is a very serious condition that can possibly lead to a fatal heart attack. Much can be done for people with this condition, however. What with the availability of medication, angioplasty, coronary stent placement, bypass surgery, and the like, it's almost criminal to avoid seeking proper medical attention.

Congestive heart failure (CHF) deserves special consideration —particularly because it is so often the cause of hospitalization in older adults. In this condition the heart muscle's pump action is weakened; it can't pump out the blood effectively. As the volume of blood it pumps out with each beat decreases, the result can be an accumulation of fluid in the lungs and other parts of the body, such as the ankles and legs—a condition called *edema*. People with severe CHF can have noticeable muscle wasting and weakness so pronounced that they are unable to perform everyday tasks.

Resistance training can dramatically improve muscle strength and functionality in these people. And endurance exercises—such as brisk walking or cycling—can improve their heart and lung function. *But remember that exercise should be avoided during flare-ups or exacerbations.* People with CHF who develop chest discomfort, shortness of breath, or a fluttering in the chest should check with their physician.

Many chronic problems are characterized by alternating periods of exacerbation and remission—periods when the disease gets better and stabilizes and periods when it worsens. While this is particularly common in congestive heart failure, it is also true of most other chronic conditions. As has been said, *exercise should only be undertaken when your condition is stable*—an important caveat for all chronic conditions. Exercise that would be enormously beneficial to an individual in a stable condition could be extremely harmful during a flare-up or a period of instability. Again, the more you know about your disease, the better. (Surely it goes without saying that anyone with a chronic condition should be under the care of a physician on a regular basis anyway.)

In general, if you're going to increase your exertion, and particularly if you're a male over 40 or a female over 50, you should first have a medical checkup. Having said that, almost everyone should be exercising on a regular basis, regardless of their age or level of fitness. (See the National Institute on Aging's recommended list of important reasons to check with your physician before starting an exercise program below.) If you're at high risk for cardiovascular disease because you're a smoker, very obese, or have a family history of heart disease or diabetes, be certain to check with your doctor before increasing your exertion.

REASONS TO CHECK WITH YOUR DOCTOR BEFORE EXERCISING
(from the National Institute on Aging)

- *any new, undiagnosed symptom*

- *chest pain*

- *irregular, rapid, or fluttery heartbeat*

- *severe shortness of breath*

- *significant, ongoing weight loss that hasn't been diagnosed*

- *infections, such as pneumonia, accompanied by fever*

- *fever itself, which can cause dehydration and a rapid heartbeat*

- *acute deep-vein thrombosis (blood clot)*

- *a hernia that is causing symptoms*

- *foot or ankle sores that won't heal*

- *joint swelling*

- *persistent pain or a disturbance in walking after you have fallen (You might have a fracture and not know it, and exercise could cause further injury.)*

- *certain eye conditions, such as bleeding in the retina or detached retina (Before you exercise after a cataract or lens implant, or after laser treatment or other eye surgery, check with your physician.)*

I believe that anyone who *can* do vigorous exercise—the vast majority of us, at any rate—*should* do vigorous exercise. Those of us who can't indulge in vigorous exercise should be involved regularly in mild to moderate exercise. Now is our chance to be that second mouse—the one that gets the cheese!

OTHER PRECAUTIONS

There are some additional precautions you need to know about. I think you should wait two hours before exercising after a meal—while your digestive system is hard at work. Knowing this, your body has directed your bloodflow toward your digestive tract. Since exercise would redirect your bloodflow to your muscles and *away* from your digestive tract, it doesn't make sense. So if you've just eaten a hearty meal, rest for at least two hours before starting to exercise.

What if you have a cold or an upper respiratory infection? Should you or should you not exercise? Some have recommended this rule-of-thumb question: *Above the chin or below the chin?* If you have a stuffy nose and a mild sore throat, it's okay to exercise. If you have fever, muscle aches, cough, or shortness of breath—don't exercise. Having said that, some studies have shown that vigorous activity increases viral replication or multiplication. So if you're feeling poorly, I recommend that you take it easy and rest until you're feeling better—regardless of whether it's above the chin or below the chin. When you do resume exercise, start off gradually. Begin with half the amount of your regular routine for half the amount of time; then gradually progress to your full routine.

WHERE TO EXERCISE

You don't have to join a gym or a health club to get exercise; you surely don't need a lot of fancy equipment. Almost all the benefits of exercise can be achieved at home. Stretching exercises, balance exercises, endurance exercises, and even strength training can be done at home. For many of these exercises, such as walking or jogging, all you need is a proper pair of shoes. If this minimal approach works for you—and if you stay with it—that's great. *But be honest with yourself.* Many of us, if not most of us, *won't* do it at home. We won't do it right; we won't do it regularly; we won't do it enough; and before long we'll get bored and stop doing it at all.

I know that many exercise facilities are noisy and can seem intimidating—populated by beautiful young girls in leotards and young studs in tank tops all strutting their fabulous figures and bulging muscles. But there are still many advantages to joining a health facility—particularly one that has special programs for mature adults. Some facilities are exclusively dedicated to mature adults (people over the age of 45). Others have dedicated hours or sessions and special programs for mature adults. In this kind of a program, you can get some individual instruction on what exercises might particularly benefit you as an individual. In other words, you can learn what your individual weaknesses are and how you can best address them with exercise. You can also learn the proper form and the best sequence of doing the different exercises and have your progress monitored more accurately. Any mistakes you're making in your exercise program can be identified and corrected more quickly. Getting this kind of help can be of great importance in preventing injury and improving results.

THE SOCIAL VALUE OF GROUP EXERCISE

The "group dynamic" is a very important success factor. At facilities like Nifty after Fifty, we encourage one another, each of us helping to motivate the other and taking pride in our collective progress. Count the benefits: It can be a ton of fun. We can enjoy each other's company on a regular basis. We can inspire others to form similar groups with a common goal: *to improve the way we feel and the way we age.* Most people find this to be a fabulous way to make new friends. Jogging clubs, gardening clubs, and neighborhood walking clubs can also be good examples of the same dynamic at work.

These clubs couple healthful activity with social interaction. If you can be involved in any of these activities, that's great. The merit of walking clubs is that they encourage exercise and togetherness. The valuable point here is that *people who play together may stay together—and stay with the program together.* On the flip side, walking groups don't differentiate the exercise needs of the individual. Some people can walk faster and for longer distances than others. It's a great exercise, but if you can do a lot more, you should do a lot more—for better fitness. Now I know that's not everyone's cup of tea. Many people enjoy exercising with more privacy, and that's okay too—if you'll do it. But these differences aside, I believe that *most of us* would be better served by starting a program at a facility like Nifty after Fifty for 8 to 16 weeks to get initiated—to learn how to do it right. Then if you choose to do all or some of your workouts at home, you'll be better trained, less prone to injury, more disciplined, and more likely to stick with it.

PERSONAL TRAINERS

For some, a personal trainer may be a fine (but expensive) idea. In selecting a personal trainer, you want to know all you can about their qualifications and experience—because almost anyone can call himself or herself a personal trainer. Licensed physical therapists usually make very good fitness trainers. Why? Because of their experience in dealing with disability and muscle weakness. Important, too, is the level of experience a prospective trainer has had with mature or older adults—and the personal compatibility or lack thereof that you perceive during an interview. Some personal trainers, for example, are overzealous about performing exercises through a full range of motion. While full range of motion is ideal, older adults may have significant limitations in this regard.

I recommend checking out your prospective trainer carefully. It could help a lot to observe him or her working with a client. Note how attentive the trainer is (or is not) to the client's activity. Are the trainer's eyes wandering about the room or engaged in conversation with someone else while the client is exercising? Don't sign up until you make a considered judgment. But make no mistake about it: A knowledgeable and attentive personal trainer can be very motivational and have a highly positive effect on your progress.

What is a knowledgeable personal trainer? As an example, one who knows the effects that certain medications might have on heart rate and blood pressure could be of great value to both the trainer and the client. In this regard, there are some excellent courses of instruction in adult and senior fitness training that are university-affiliated or sponsored by the American College of Sports Medicine. Some fitness organizations and clubs also sponsor excellent programs. But be aware that there are other fitness clubs that certify trainers after as little as 48 hours of instruction! So it's really important that you be diligent in your inquiry as to a prospective trainer's qualifications.

In my opinion, a licensing test or examination that would certify candidates as adult and senior fitness trainers would go a long way toward establishing a baseline level of qualifications and competency. I hope that becomes available in the not too distant future.

FREQUENCY OF EXERCISE

The ideal frequency and type of exercise is going to vary from one individual to another. But let me give you some general guidelines. I think you should do stretching exercises every day, and strength, balance, and endurance training two or three days a week. Your individual level of fitness or unfitness will be an important determinant. Some of us will exercise two or three times a week by combining strength and endurance training.

Others will want to work out seven days a week. For example: You might do strength and balance training on Mondays, Wednesdays, and Fridays and switch to endurance training on Tuesdays, Thursdays, and Saturdays. On Sundays you might only do stretching—a daily exercise. A seven-day program may sound gruesome to some of you who haven't gotten started yet. But believe me—when you get into it, you'll feel so much better you won't know yourself. You'll love it!

After you get started and feel confident that you're on your way, you'll be able to do some of the workouts at home—such as balance and stretching exercises. But in my opinion, the strength-training program can more effectively and more safely be done two or three times a week with supervision, and more often than not, with the use of specific resistance machines. By this means, a safe range of motion and the proper form can be individually established and imprinted on your mind. Strength training can also be adjusted to encompass a cardiopulmonary workout. Some people can achieve an excellent level of fitness this way and only work out two or three days a week.

Just imagine it! You can get stronger. You can improve your balance, your flexibility, and your mental acuity. You can improve your endurance and the quality of your life. You can enhance the way you look and feel. Just *think about it!* You can accomplish all of this with 20- to 30-minute workouts two to three times a week. Regardless of whether you're 50 or 90 years old, *you can be Nifty after Fifty.* So how about it? Grab your designer sweat suit, or just come as you are—and let's get it on!

LOOKING BACK, LOOKING FORWARD

CHAPTER 11 REVIEW ◆ ◆ ◆

◆ No matter how old you are, a program of regular physical exercise can be of enormous benefit to your ongoing quality of life.

◆ As physical exercise increases your strength and endurance, it also improves the function of your brain, heart, lungs, gastrointestinal tract, and metabolism.

◆ Muscle weakness, a primary cause of frailty, can be halted and even reversed by a regular program of strength training.

◆ Certain chronic health problems must be thoroughly discussed with your doctor before undertaking any vigorous exercise.

CHAPTER 12 PREVIEW ◆ ◆ ◆

◆ Why is it important to do a little stretching both before and after a workout?

◆ What happens to our muscles, tendons, and ligaments as we grow older? Can exercise improve our range of motion and make us less prone to injury?

◆ Are there special exercises to improve flexibility in specific body parts such as the neck and shoulders? How about the back, arms, and legs?

◆ Why is it a good idea to use the "buddy system" when exercising on the floor?

12

STRETCHING

*A muscle is like a car. If you want it to run well
early in the morning, you have to warm it up.*
—Florence Griffith-Joyner

Blessed are the flexible, for they shall not be bent out of shape.
—Sue Petrie Marsha

It's true that stretching may not burn many calories or increase your strength and endurance. But believe me, stretching movements can make the rest of your exercise program much more effective and enjoyable—and they only take about five minutes! It's a fact that as we get older, our bodies get stiffer. Our flexibility and range of motion decrease. When we exceed that limited range of motion, we can easily tear or strain our muscle and ligament fibers, which causes injury and pain. These injuries can interrupt our exercise program and put us on the sidelines, and on some occasions they can be quite serious.

Stretching improves flexibility by preventing the tightening of muscles and freezing of joints. As we age, muscles and tendons tend to tighten, and ligaments often undergo increasing fibrosis. This may make them harder, less elastic—even calcified. Together with arthritic changes in the joints, this tightening process leaves us less flexible and more prone to injury. Can you identify with the following common situations? Say we pull something in our backs when we bend over, or in our shoulders when we lift something. Even worse, perhaps we aren't able to avoid an oncoming car when we're driving. Why? Because we can't turn to look in both directions very well. And when we twist an ankle or fall, we have a greater likelihood of tearing ligaments or developing a fracture—all because of a lack of flexibility.

All that said—what's the difference between a tendon and a ligament? Let me explain: A tendon is that part of the muscle that attaches to and moves the bone when the muscle contracts. This illustration is an example of the biceps muscle—the big muscle in the front of your upper arm. Notice that it attaches to the shoulder and the forearm. This muscle contracts and shortens to bend your arm.

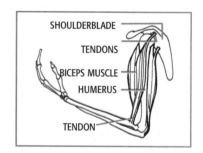

Ligaments, on the other hand, are firm fibrous structures that support the various joints in our body. The illustration on the left below depicts a joint with healthy, elastic ligaments undergoing flexion. The illustration on the right depicts a joint with a sclerotic or hardened ligament undergoing similar flexion.

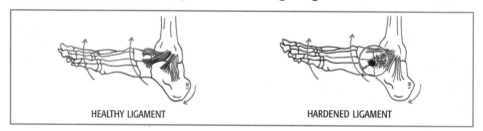

As you can see, the joint with the sclerotic ligament, being less elastic, tends to tear some of its fibers—and even a piece of bone. How about that! The less elastic ligaments tore and caused a fracture.

So now we know that a lack of flexibility due to tight tendons and sclerotic ligaments can have many important consequences. It increases your chance of sprains, torn ligaments, fractures, and muscle strains. It decreases your range of motion (how far you can move your arms, legs, neck, or any part of your body in different directions). During exercise, a decreased range of motion equates to a decrease in the actual exercise—simply because you're moving your limbs a shorter distance. That's why I believe that if you stretch for life, you just might stretch your life—but let's get there gradually.

THE PRINCIPLES OF STRETCHING EXERCISES

Before getting into the specifics of each exercise, let me share some important concepts that apply to all stretching exercises. I think mild stretching *before* a workout is a good idea—but warm up first with a little walking and by swinging your arms. Why? Because stretching cold muscles can sometimes result in injury. Then, after a workout, your muscles are pumped and tight. That's why it's important to do some stretching at the *end* of each exercise session.

Please note that stretching is not a competitive sport. If the guy next to you can touch his toes and you can't—so what? *Your* goal is to improve your own flexibility—or even more importantly, to prevent it from decreasing as you age.

All movements should be slow and deliberate—not jerky. And each stretch should be maintained for 15 to 30 seconds and then repeated two to four more times. Don't rush through the stretching maneuvers. Stretch slowly, and *slightly* bend your joints—don't lock them. If you're experiencing pain in the course of a stretch, then you're pushing too far. Stretching exercises should not be painful. If a particular movement starts to hurt, back off a little and stretch to a point just short of the pain. Over a period of weeks, very gradually increase your stretch with each movement. If you follow these principles on a regular basis, you will achieve a new and flexible you! Now strive to maintain this new and wonderful level of flexibility by stretching at least three times a week—preferably every day.

Check with your physician if you've had hip, knee, back, or any other kind of major orthopedic surgery. Certain types of stretching exercises might not be a good choice for you. As an example, if you've had a hip replacement, you shouldn't bend your hips more than 90 degrees or cross your legs.

FLOOR EXERCISES AND THE BUDDY SYSTEM

Many stretching exercises are done on the floor. Special care has to be taken if you've had hip replacement surgery or if you have a bad back. Some people are hesitant to lie down on the floor. Why? They're afraid they may have difficulty getting back up! Any of you who have this concern should use a buddy system for floor exercises—someone who can assist you in getting up and down. What should you do in the absence of a buddy? You can safely get down and back up from a prone position by a series of movements as follows:

(1) Put your hands on the seat of a sturdy chair.

(2) Lower yourself down on one knee.

(3) Bring the other knee down.

(4) Put one hand on the floor and leave the other hand on the seat of the chair as you lower yourself onto your hip.

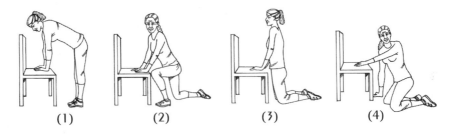

(1)   (2)   (3)   (4)

(5) Now you are lying on your side with your weight on your hip.

(6) From this position, roll over onto your back.

(7) To get up, first roll back onto your side. Then place your hands on the floor at about the level of your upper chest.

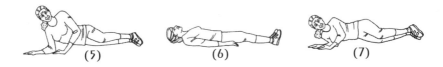

(5)   (6)   (7)

(8) Now push your shoulders off the floor. While leaning on your hands for support, shift your weight in the direction of your knees so that you are on all fours.

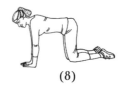

(8)

(9)   Then place your hands on the seat of the chair, and lift one of your legs so that your foot is flat on the floor.

(10) Now rise up, using both legs and the hands you've placed on the seat of the chair.

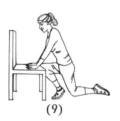
(9)

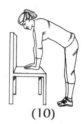
(10)

NECK-STRETCHING EXERCISES

It's a good idea to be seated comfortably in a straight-back chair when doing neck-stretching exercises. For some exercises, you can lie on the floor, knees bent, with a firm pillow beneath your head. It's really important to do these exercises slowly. Why? Because sudden changes in the position of the head can cause dizziness—particularly in people who have inner ear problems. Be sure to avoid a bouncing motion. Also, if you've had any neck or back problems, be sure to get your doctor's okay before trying these exercises.

To loosen the back of your neck, begin by slowly bending your head forward. Try to put your chin on your chest until you feel a pleasant stretching sensation in the back of your neck.

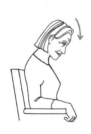

Hold this position for 15 seconds before slowly returning your head to the upright position. Then repeat the exercise three or four times. Straighten up slowly between each movement. (Do not jerk your head.)

To loosen the front of your neck, slowly bend your head back to look up at the ceiling until you feel a pleasant stretching sensation in the front of your neck. To avoid *leaning* backward, do this exercise in a chair with a supportive straight back. Hold this position 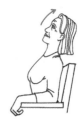 for 10 to 15 seconds before slowly returning to the resting position. Repeat the movement three to five times. Don't rush. Each time you are at your full stretch, open and close your mouth slowly to count the seconds, and hum a *mmm* sound each time you close your mouth for a second. This will also help to stretch the tissues in the front of your neck. Repeat this two more times.

Now for the sides of your neck: Look straight ahead. Tilt your head toward one shoulder and then toward the other shoulder. As always, do this slowly and hold the stretch for 10 to 20 seconds. Repeat the movement three to five times. It's a good idea to do this movement in front of a mirror. That will help you avoid raising or shrugging your shoulder toward your head. The object is not to touch the side of your head with your shoulder. Your goal is simply to stretch the side of your neck opposite the direction that you're tilting your head. And remember— no jerking motions!

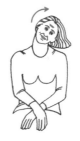
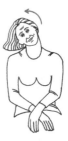

NECK ROTATION

You can do neck rotation exercises by (1) lying on the floor with a firm pillow or a book under your head, or (2) sitting with your head in a level position, neither looking down nor looking up. Start by

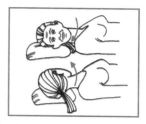

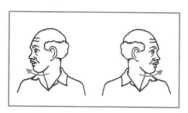

turning your head first to the left as far as it will go—just to a level of mild discomfort. Hold it there for 15 seconds. Now go back to the forward viewing position and turn your head very slowly to the right. Hold it there for 15 seconds. Then turn back again to the forward viewing position. Repeat this two or three more times.

The last neck-stretching exercise combines all the neck stretches into one slow-moving stretch. It's a very slow rotation. The starting position is looking down, with your chin on your chest. Rotate your head very slowly all the way to the right. Continue the rotation by bringing your head back so that you're looking at the ceiling, then onto your left shoulder, and finally all the way down to the starting position (with your chin on your chest). Then do the same rotation in the other direction. Moving slowly, repeat this two or three more times in each direction.

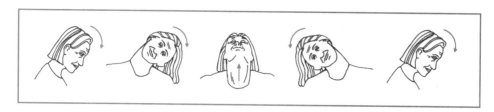

Don't be alarmed if you hear snapping or popping sounds. These are common in stretching exercises, but they're not dangerous. If you have a medical history of neck problems, however, check with your doctor before doing these exercises. The important thing to remember is this: *Don't stretch to the point of causing pain.* Always stretch slowly and deliberately.

STRETCHING THE ARMS AND SHOULDERS

All you need is a towel to perform marvelous exercises that stretch the muscles and the ligaments of the upper arms, shoulders, and elbows. Holding the towel with your right hand, bend your elbow and drape the towel down your back. Then grasp the towel with your left hand behind your back. Now gradually grasp the towel higher and higher with your left hand. The resulting downward movement of your right hand toward your left hand stretches your triceps, shoulders, and elbows. Hold this position for 10–20 seconds and then reverse your hands.

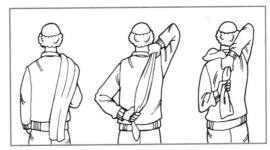

Remember to stretch only until it's a little bit uncomfortable, but not to the point of pain. Avoiding any jerky motions, hold the stretch for 10 to 20 seconds. Now reverse your hands so that your left hand is on top. Put your right hand behind your back to grasp the lower end of the towel. Gradually inch your hands closer and closer together until you feel a mild stretching sensation in your shoulders, upper arms, and elbows. Repeat this two more times and hold each stretch for 10 to 20 seconds. See how much more limber you feel!

Now lie down on a mat in front of your chair—head held straight on a pillow and knees slightly bent. (Use the techniques

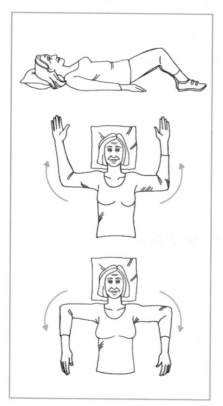

described earlier for getting into the lying position.) Stretch your arms straight out to the side, and then bend them at the elbow so your hands are pointing toward the ceiling. (Keep your shoulders and elbows flat on the floor and your arms bent at 90 degrees throughout this exercise.) Now let your hands and forearms slowly roll backward from the elbow so that your fingers are pointing toward your head. As soon as you feel a stretch or slight discomfort—that's where you stop. Don't try to stretch too far or too fast. Slowly raise your hands and forearms, still bending your elbows, and point your fingers toward the ceiling again. Then let your arms slowly roll forward, remaining bent at the elbow, to point toward your toes. Maintain each position for 10 to 20 seconds. Repeat the movements three to five times.

WRISTS AND HANDS

While sitting in a chair, you can stretch your wrists and hands. Simply put your hands together in front of your chest as if you were praying. Keep the heels of your hands and 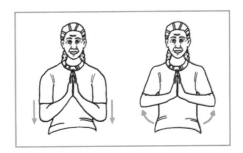 your fingertips together. Then slowly raise your elbows while keeping your hands together. You'll feel a slight stretching sensation in your wrists and in your fingers. Hold it for 10–30 seconds, then relax for a few seconds. Repeat this movement two or three more times.

STRETCHING THE OUTER THIGHS AND HIPS

Get back on the floor to stretch the muscles of your thighs and hips. *(If you've had hip surgery or hip or knee problems, don't do this exercise unless your physician approves it.)* The starting position is on your back with a pillow under your head. Keep your knees bent and together, and keep your shoulders and feet flat on the floor.

Gently rotate your knees, first to the right side as far as possible without causing pain—just until you feel a mild stretch. Hold this position for about 15 seconds, and go back to the

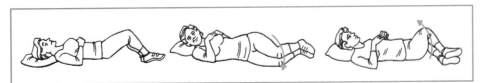

starting position. Then rotate your knees to the left side until you feel a mild stretch. Hold that position for 15 seconds. Repeat the movement two or three more times to each side, holding the stretch for 15 to 20 seconds each time.

QUADRICEPS STRETCH

The quadriceps are the muscles in the front of your thighs. *(Again, if you've had hip or knee problems, please check with* 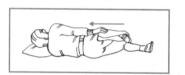 *your physician before doing this exercise.)* To stretch these muscles, first roll onto your left side. Bend your right leg at the knee and grasp your foot with your right hand. If you can't reach your foot, extend your reach by looping a towel (or clasped belt) over the top of your right foot. Then, gently pull on the towel until you feel a mild stretching sensation in the front of your right knee and thigh. Hold the stretch for 15 to 20 seconds before rolling onto your right side and repeating the movement. Do this two or three times on each side. This maneuver can also be effective in stretching the front of your ankle.

STRETCHING THE INNER THIGHS

Again, if you've had hip or knee problems, talk with your doctor before doing this exercise. The starting position for this movement is lying flat on your back. Bend your right knee upward toward your head. Then, moving your knee in a sideways direction, slowly lower it toward the floor. When you feel a mild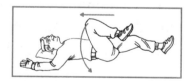

stretch, hold it for about 15 seconds. Then return to the starting position by bringing your knee slowly back into place. Repeat this again with each leg two or three times, and hold the stretch for 15 seconds each time. Keep your shoulders, back, hips, and pelvis flat on the floor throughout this stretch.

STRETCHING THE BACK OF THE THIGHS

This exercise will stretch your hamstrings—the muscles in the back of your thigh. *(Once again, if you've had hip problems, you should check with your physician before doing these exercises.)* Sit sideways on a bench and stretch out one leg on the bench. The other leg is off the bench with your foot flat on the floor. Don't try to lock the leg on the bench; it doesn't have to be absolutely straight.

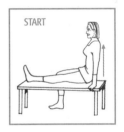

Gradually—very gradually—bend forward at the hips, not at the waist. When you feel a mild stretching sensation in the back of your leg, hold it there for 15 seconds and then relax. Don't cause yourself any pain. Repeat this movement two or three more times with each leg.

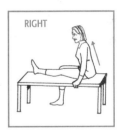

To get maximum benefit from this exercise, the foot that's on the floor should be kept flat, and your shoulders should be kept straight throughout the movement. Be sure to move slowly without any jerking motions.

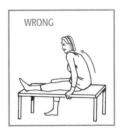

For those of you who don't have a bench at home, here's an alternative method of doing a hamstring stretch using a straight-back chair. Hold the back of the chair with both hands, and bend forward from the hips (not your waist). Keep your back and shoulders straight throughout the entire maneuver—until your

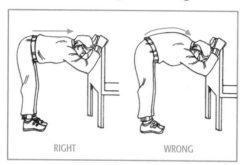

RIGHT   WRONG

upper body is parallel to the floor. Again, hold this position for 15 seconds, and repeat the movement three to five times. Do this stretch slowly, without jerking or humping your back.

STRETCHING OUR CALF MUSCLES

To stretch the calf muscles, stand facing a wall. Place your palms flat against the wall. Then step back with one foot about one to two feet. Stand with both knees slightly bent, and keep your back foot flat on the floor. Now gradually straighten your back knee *while keeping your front knee slightly bent.* When

you feel a pleasant stretch in the back of your calf, hold that position for about 15 seconds. Then do the same routine with the other leg. Repeat this movement with each leg two or three more times.

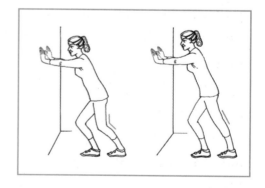

BACK-STRETCHING MOVEMENTS

Many of us get up each morning with a sore back. This is often the result of a bad mattress or at least a poorly supportive one. A firmer, more supportive mattress could go a long way toward solving this problem. Some have even found it beneficial to put a bed board made of 3/4-inch plywood under the mattress. Others, however, have found it necessary to get a mattress with a greater degree of segmental support. If chronic low-back pain is a problem, you might try sleeping on your back instead of your abdomen. Place a pillow under your knees. This will help you keep your knees slightly bent and reduce the tension on your low-back muscles.

You can often loosen your stiff and aching back muscles right at your bedside before you get up. Sit on the side of your bed with your feet flat on the floor. Then gradually bend at the hips (not at the waist) by dropping your shoulders and extending your arms forward between your knees. Hold your hands palm down and bend forward until you feel a pleasant stretching sensation in your lower back. Hold the stretch for 10 to 15 seconds. You don't have to touch the floor, but as your flexibility improves, you may actually be able to put the palms of your hands flat on the floor. Do this movement slowly and repeat it two or three times.

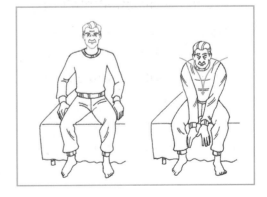

You can do the same kind of low-back stretch in a chair. Fold your arms in front of your chest. Then let your shoulders and head bend forward. As your head drops between your 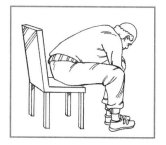 knees, you should feel a mild stretching in your lower back. Hold the stretch for 10 to 15 seconds. Remember to bend mostly at the hips, not the waist. Go back to the starting position and repeat this movement two or three more times.

MORE BACK STRETCHING

Lie on your back with a pillow under your head and your knees bent. Keeping your shoulders flat and your knees together, clasp your hands around your bent knees. Gently pull your knees toward your chest, and hold this stretch for 10 to 15 seconds before returning to the starting position. Repeat the movement two or three more times.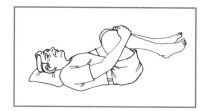

YOUR BACK AND YOUR ABS

Most people don't realize that there's a secret to maintaining a healthy back. *The secret is to maintain good abdominal muscle tone.* This can't be emphasized enough. Well-toned abdominal muscles decrease the drag on your lower back. Look for more information on strengthening the abdominal muscles in the next two chapters.

But, while you're still on your back, here's one exercise I'd like you to try. It's called the *flat back position.* As the name implies, the starting position is flat on your back, with your knees bent and your feet flat on the floor. Try to tighten your abdominal muscles and your buttocks at the same time. This movement tends to flatten your back against the mat or floor. It may require some concentration and coordination to get the hang of it—but once you get it, it will be both a good abdominal and a good back exercise for you. Hold it for five seconds and repeat it two or three times.

LOOKING BACK, LOOKING FORWARD

CHAPTER 12 REVIEW ◆ ◆ ◆

◆ Slow and steady stretching exercises are a crucial component of an overall exercise program.

◆ Regular, focused stretching movements improve flexibility, increase range of motion, and prevent injury.

◆ People who have had any orthopedic surgery or problems should talk with their doctor before starting stretching exercises.

◆ Specific stretching exercises can reduce stiffness in the neck, arms and shoulders, wrists and hands, hips and thighs, calves, back, and abs.

CHAPTER 13 PREVIEW ◆ ◆ ◆

◆ Why is it so important to improve the strength and tone of your muscles—even if you don't want to be a bodybuilder?

◆ What advantages might resistance training machines have over free weights? What kinds of machines are there, and how do they work?

◆ Why are correct form and proper breathing technique so important to an effective strength-training program?

◆ Is it true that contracting and stretching muscles actually has a positive effect on your brain chemistry?

13

STRENGTH TRAINING

Lack of activity destroys the good condition of every human being, while movement and methodical exercise save it and preserve it.

—Plato

Why is it important to have visible stomach muscles? I grew up in an era (the Paleolithic) when people kept their stomach muscles discreetly out of sight.

—Sue Petrie Marsha

What happens when you contract and stretch a muscle against resistance? Every fiber in that muscle can be called into play. Then, as the muscle fatigues, a pleasant sensation much like an internal massage is produced, followed by release of endorphins that makes you feel great. In fact, as I've said earlier, those endorphins can actually addict you to exercise and really make you feel more *alive*!

Most of us have heard the old saw about resistance training: *no pain, no gain.* Well, I'm here to tell you that it doesn't have to hurt—and that, in fact, it *shouldn't* hurt. As you exercise a muscle, it becomes fatigued, tight, and pumped with blood. This causes a soothing, warm sensation or a slight burn in the muscle. It's common to experience some mild muscle soreness after a strength-training workout but nothing like real pain—unless you're overdoing it. Resting the muscle and repeating the exercise process is the way you build the strength and tone of the muscle.

The best part is that the results of resistance training come quickly. You'll be much stronger in just eight weeks. In fact, you might become as strong as, or even stronger than, you were 20 years ago!

A caution: *It's extremely important to maintain proper form while doing resistance exercises.* Proper form prevents injury and ensures that you get the maximum benefit from each repetition. Mirrors, while not essential, can also help serve your purpose. Why? Because by watching yourself as you exercise, you can better monitor and correct your form.

PNEUMATICS, VARIABLE RESISTANCE, AND INERTIA

The law of inertia is one of the simplest laws of physics. In a nutshell: *Things at rest tend to stay at rest, and things in motion tend to stay in motion.* That's why it requires more effort to start a weight in motion than to keep it moving. You know—it's easier to push a car with a dead battery after it has started rolling than it is to get it moving from a dead stop—and it's also harder to *stop* it after it's moving.

The same is true with moving weight in resistance exercises. It requires more power to get the weight moving from the starting position than to keep it moving. And it also takes more effort to stop it when returning to the starting position. That's why I believe that starting the weight in motion and stopping the weight on the return can cause some muscle and ligamentous disruption or damage. When this results in pain, it decreases the effectiveness and enjoyment of your exercise. It may even cause negative psychological feedback that discourages exercise altogether.

The question is: Are there resistance-training machines that can effectively deal with this problem? Fortunately, there are a couple of solutions.

Pneumatic machines, such as those made by the Keiser Corp., are among my favorites. That's why we use them at our Nifty after Fifty centers. With pneumatic machines, the resistance you push or pull against is air pressure—which is easily increased or decreased by using conveniently placed control buttons. More importantly, the resistance is linear rather than influenced by inertia. This system allows you to smoothly and quietly increase your strength *while avoiding the potentially injurious effects of inertia.*

Another solution is the use of "variable resistance" machines. With this kind of equipment, the weight-resistance at the starting point of each exercise is considerably less than the weight-resistance at the midpoint of the exercise. The machines are engineered to gradually increase the resistance from the starting point to the midpoint of the movement. The idea is that your muscles have less power at the starting point and are stronger at the midpoint of the movement. This should decrease the stress on joints and muscle fibers that can be caused by inertia.

So, wherever you go to exercise, try to use exercise machines that reduce the effects of inertia.

FREE WEIGHTS

Free weights are wonderful. You can get a great workout and build enormous strength by using them. Professional bodybuilders and competitive weightlifters use free weights extensively. But you must be aware that they can subject your joints and muscles to the effects of inertia. That's why there's a tendency to swing the weight and cheat on form. So when you use free weights, even greater diligence as to maintaining form is essential. Despite this caveat, some exercises are actually *best* performed with free weights. Nonetheless, it's best to develop a reasonable level of fitness with weight machines before using free weights too much.

The bottom line: Regardless of the type of resistance training you choose—free weights, pneumatic resistance, or weight machines—you can get very strong, very toned, very well-defined, and even very big, but only if you want to.

REPS AND SETS

The jargon of resistance training comes down to two terms: *reps* and *sets*. The term "rep" is short for *repetition*—meaning the performance of an exercise movement from the starting position through the range of motion and back to the starting position. The *positive phase* of each rep consists of moving against the resistance or weight from the starting position to the end point of the exercise movement. The *negative phase* consists of returning the weight-resistance back to the starting position. Equally important, both phases of the rep should be done slowly, deliberately, and with perfect form. Both the positive and negative phases are exercising and strengthening your muscles.

Just remember this: *Slow, lighter, and in good form is better than quick, heavy, and sloppy.* The positive phase of each rep should be done to a count of two, and the negative phase to the count of four. This simple trick may work for some of you: Use the word *repetition* (a four-syllable word) along with the term "rep" to count your reps and to do each rep to the proper count.

For example, count to yourself—REP-ONE during the positive phase of the movement and RE-PE-TI-TION ONE during the negative phase. Then count REP-TWO for the positive phase of the second rep and RE-PE-TI-TION TWO for the negative phase of the second rep—and so on until you have completed the number of reps in the "set" (the number of consecutive reps that you do of any one exercise). The number of reps in a set may vary from as little as three to as many as 20. Generally, however, a set will consist of 8 to 15 reps. The number of sets for any one exercise may vary from one to five. Rest periods between each set may vary from 45 seconds to two and a half minutes.

It's important to approach new exercise routines gradually. Each of us will progress at a different rate and have a different level of tolerance (in terms of how much we can or even how much we *should* do). The important thing is that all of us will improve by sticking to it. Even more exciting is the fact that this improvement will be obvious in six to eight weeks—and you'll love it.

It's important to breathe easily throughout the exercise movements. At the beginning of each exercise, take a deep breath. Then, as you perform the positive movement against resistance, exhale to the count of two. The exhalation should be completed at the same time you complete the positive phase of each rep. As you perform the negative phase of each rep by returning to the starting position, you should inhale and fill your lungs with air. Each repetition is performed in the same manner. This sounds very easy—but it's even easier to do it incorrectly! So concentrate on developing this pattern throughout your entire exercise session. You'll be surprised at how soon it will become second nature to you.

ABOUT BREATHING

There's a natural tendency to hold your breath when doing resistance training. But that's the wrong thing to do. Because breathing is extremely important, let's take a moment to go over the basics. There are two phases to breathing: *inhaling* (taking the air into your lungs) and *exhaling* (expelling the air from your lungs). What happens as you inhale? Your diaphragm, the large muscle that separates your chest from your abdomen, descends. As your diaphragm contracts and descends, your *glottis*, the entrance into your windpipe or trachea, is open. The descent of the diaphragm results in a negative pressure within your chest—much like a bellows. This negative pressure causes your lungs to expand as the air flows into your trachea. In the back of your throat a flap called the *epiglottis* protects the glottis (the

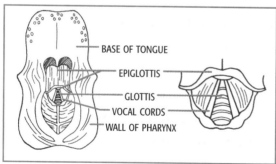

BASE OF TONGUE

EPIGLOTTIS

GLOTTIS

VOCAL CORDS

WALL OF PHARYNX

opening to your trachea) by preventing food and other unwanted material from entering your windpipe. The epiglottis opens and closes the glottis as you inhale and exhale air. So in order for you to hold your breath, the epiglottis, as shown in this illustration, closes over the opening (the glottis) to the trachea.

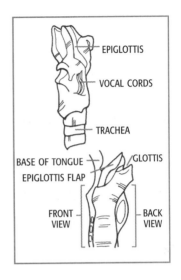

As a side note, this is what many of you can do when you strain to lift something or try to force a hard bowel movement. You take a deep breath and force an exhalation against a closed glottis. This is called the *Valsalva maneuver*. Basically, it consists of a forced exhalation against a closed airway (the glottis closed by the epiglottis). When you perform this grunting Valsalva maneuver, you dramatically increase the pressure within your chest. This raises your blood pressure and increases the pressure on all the organs and blood vessels in your chest.

In contrast, you do this more gently when you're swimming underwater or anytime you hold your breath. But when you do this too forcefully, you're compressing your internal organs and producing an adverse effect on your circulatory system. Exactly how does this play out? When the pressure on the major veins in your chest is increased, it slows the return of blood from the rest of your body to your chest and heart. Since your heart is receiving less blood, each beat has less blood to pump out to the very muscles we're exercising. Although this is the type of straining used by some professional bodybuilders and competitive weight-lifters, it's *not* what your training program should be about!

THE PRINCIPLES OF RESISTANCE TRAINING

Determining the "max" and the proper exercise resistance

The principles of using resistance machines or free weights are the same in terms of reps, sets, and rest periods. You must be correctly positioned and maintain proper form and breathing techniques while performing each exercise.

First, perform the movement on each machine with no resistance. This will help you establish the correct form for each movement as well as the proper range of motion. Then, warm up by using a very slight amount of resistance for five to eight repetitions. After resting approximately two minutes, increase the resistance for five repetitions, and then rest again for approximately two minutes. Now try to see how much resistance you can tolerate as you perform the movement *once*. For practical purposes we will call this your *maximum effort*—also referred to as your "max" for that exercise. Be sure that you're not holding your breath in performing this maximum movement; breathe properly, as previously discussed.

Then, having determined your maximum effort, use 70 to 75 percent of this resistance for your exercises. Repeat this procedure with each machine or exercise. Examples: If your max on one machine or exercise is 100 pounds, use 70 to 75 pounds to exercise on that machine, and do five to eight reps with that resistance. If your max on another machine is 80 pounds, use 60 pounds. If your max on still another machine is 40 pounds, use 30 pounds to do five to eight reps. Each time you do an exercise, perform five to eight repetitions with perfect form. Rest between sets. To build muscle mass, many experts recommend that the rest period between sets should be two and a half minutes in order to clear most of the lactate from your muscles. Later in this chapter we'll discuss some variations—depending on your conditioning and whether or not you want to combine cardiopulmonary conditioning with your resistance training program.

As you become stronger, you might do only one set of each exercise or as many as two to eight sets at each station. Gradually, as your conditioning improves, you can increase the number of reps to 8 or 15 and the number of sets to three or five, while at the same time decreasing the rest periods between sets. This should be done slowly over a period of weeks, not days. The last rep of the last set should be the most difficult. It should make you feel as if you can't do one more rep; you're just plain out of gas. When it *doesn't* feel that way—when it feels as if you've still got fuel in your tank—*the message is that you've become stronger*—so it's time for you to progress to the next step. But remember to take it gradually. Today is the first day of the rest of your life—there's no rush.

Increasing the reps and the resistance

The next step consists of increasing the number of reps in each set—perhaps to 10 and then to 12 or more. When this step is achieved, you can increase the weight-resistance and start with eight reps in each set again—because you've become stronger. Isn't that great? Just make the effort and it *will* happen to you— believe me.

Frequency of training sessions

For some of you, one set of each exercise two or three times a week will be sufficient. But many of you will want to progress to three to five sets. Most people benefit from strength training two to four times a week, but some enjoy a workout almost every day. If you exercise every day, it's important that you avoid exercising the same muscles every day. One day you might work your upper body and the next, your lower body. It might surprise you to know that your muscles become stronger while you're resting, not while you're exercising. All of the biochemical reactions that strength training calls into play (that make your muscles stronger) take about 48 hours to produce their effects. That's why you want to work different muscles on alternate days or do a complete strength-training workout two to three days a week, alternating with endurance training three days a week. Do you remember what kind of exercise should be done *daily*? That's right—*stretching exercises.*

◆ ◆ ◆

A word to the wise: Don't let strength training become an ego game. It's easy for this to occur. But if you attempt to increase the resistance too rapidly, you can hurt yourself. Most of us can move more resistance by throwing caution to the wind. We can do this by not adhering to the proper form for an exercise or by holding our breath too hard. This multiplies the chance of injury *and* limits the benefit of the exercise. It can't be said too often, so I'll say it again and again: *Whatever you do, progress gradually with good form and proper breathing techniques.*

MACHINES TO GET YOU STARTED

To start with, use a group of 10 resistance exercises that I believe will produce good fitness in all of the major muscle groups.

- **seated bench press**—exercises your chest muscles, shoulder muscles, and the triceps muscle in the back of your arm

- **seated shoulder press or vertical press**—exercises your shoulder muscles, upper back muscles, and triceps

- **triceps machine**—exercises your triceps

- **arm curl machine**—exercises your biceps and other muscles in the front of your arm

- **seated leg press**—exercises the muscles in your thigh and calf

- **seated leg curl machine**—exercises the muscles in the back of your thigh (hamstrings)

- **seated leg extension machine**—exercises the muscles in the front of your thigh (quadriceps)

- **upper back machine**—exercises the muscles of your upper back, shoulders, and arms

- **upper pull-down machine or lat bar**—exercises the mid and lower latissimus dorsi muscle

- **abdominal crunch machine**—exercises your abdominal muscles

With a few exceptions (that we'll discuss later), the principles of good strength training on all of these machines are the same. *When your strength has improved so that three sets of eight repetitions of any movement are easily performed, you can increase the number of repetitions in each set.* After increasing the number of reps from 8 to 10, 12, or possibly even more, increase the resistance. Each time you increase the resistance, go back to doing eight repetitions. As you get stronger, you can increase the number of repetitions in each set to 12 or more with this new and slightly greater resistance—and so on. When you're satisfied that you've reached a good level of fitness, you will have established your individual maintenance program. That's the workout you will be doing two or four times a week.

WARM UP AND COOL DOWN

There are a few more important points that should be emphasized. Warming up is one of them, and cooling down is another. Before starting your workout, do your stretching exercises and warm up the muscles you're going to be exercising. This can be accomplished by doing five to eight reps with half or less of the resistance you're going to use for your workout. Then, when you've completed your entire workout on all of the machines, you should cool down rather than stop cold. This can usually be accomplished by walking briskly for a few minutes and then at a slower pace for a few minutes. Then do your stretching exercises.

PRE-FATIGUE

An efficient and time-saving method of working out is to exercise muscles that are already partially worked out by a prior movement. After working out your chest, shoulders, and triceps on the seated bench press, it would save time to move on to the seated shoulder press to work out your shoulders and triceps. Having partially fatigued some of the same muscles with one exercise, you may be able to get an excellent workout on the second machine with a lesser number of reps or sets—without sacrificing any benefit. Having pre-fatigued your triceps with the first two exercises, you might then do specific triceps exercises. This way, you can effectively work out your triceps with less resistance and perhaps with a lesser number of reps or sets.

The same can be said for the seated leg press, leg extension, and leg curl machines—all of which exercise your thigh muscles. Similarly, the upper back machine and the lat pull-down machine primarily exercise your upper back and shoulders. But they also exercise and can pre-fatigue your biceps and the other muscles in the front of your arm. So using these machines prior to doing arm curls might allow you to get a good biceps workout with a lesser number of arm curl exercises.

VARIETY

To avoid muscle boredom, after a good level of fitness has been established, you should try to vary your workout. Try different machines and different exercises, and vary the sequence of the exercises. You might alter the number of reps or sets and finish off with light weight concentration reps. These are done very slowly while concentrating on tightening the muscle you're exercising. You might like the pec-deck to better isolate and exercise your

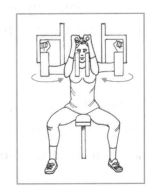

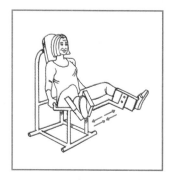

chest muscles, or the inner and outer thigh machines. Exercising the same muscles with different movements has the potential to further enhance the fitness of a muscle or group of muscles. For the first eight weeks, however, get fit on the 10 important machines mentioned.

LET'S GET STARTED

The basic principles described above are similar and applicable to all of these machines. Start by following these steps to determine your max:

STEP 1: Establish the proper form and breathing technique and the correct range of motion by doing the exercise or movement with no added resistance.

STEP 2: Warm up your muscles by doing five reps with minimal resistance and then rest for two and a half minutes.

STEP 3: Increase the resistance, and then do another five reps before resting again for two and a half minutes.

STEP 4: Try to "max"—discover the maximum amount of weight-resistance you can move through the exercise movement while using perfect form and without holding your breath. Then rest for two and a half minutes. Avoid temptation. It's true that you might be able to move a lot more resistance by holding your breath or ignoring proper form—but that's not what I want you to do.

Now you are ready to start your resistance-training program by following these steps:

STEP 1: Use 70 to 75 percent of your max to start your strength-training program. After you warm up, do five to eight reps for your first set with this resistance. Then rest for two and a half minutes.

STEP 2: Try to do a second and then a third set with this resistance, resting two and a half minutes between sets.

STEP 3: When comfortable, increase the number of reps to eight or more in each set and increase the number of sets to three.

STEP 4: As your fitness improves, try to decrease the resting period between sets to an average of two minutes.

STEP 5: The last rep of the last set should be the most difficult. If you feel you can do more, increase the number of reps in each set to 10 or 12 or more.

STEP 6: When you can do three sets of 12 or more reps for four or more consecutive workouts, increase the weight resistance slightly and go back to doing eight reps for three sets.

STEP 7: When you are satisfied with your new level of strength or find it too difficult to further increase the resistance or the number of reps or sets, you have established your maintenance. Use this level as your maintenance program for each exercise, two to four times a week. Having said this, your exercise program may be interrupted by travel or illness, making your maintenance workout harder to maintain. Not to worry. In chapter 15 we'll address some simple tricks to manage this.

But before proceeding any further, a word of caution worth repeating: To reach your goal of greater fitness, do not lose sight of these important ABCs:

A – *use perfect form with every movement*

B – *perfect the technique of proper breathing*

C – *progress gradually*

THE SEATED BENCH OR CHEST PRESS MACHINE

The seated bench press strengthens the pectoralis muscles—you know, your "pecs," or the muscles in your chest. It also strengthens your shoulder muscles and your triceps. Make sure you're positioned properly. Check that your rear end is back on the seat; don't let it slide forward. Your back should be straight and firmly positioned against the back support. Adjust the height of the seat so that the bench press handles are below your shoulders and about at the level of your upper chest. Now do a few reps with no resistance so that you get the idea of the movement—including a clear understanding of the proper form and the right way to breathe.

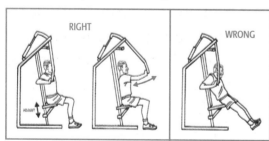

On some of the newer versions of these seated bench press machines, you'll notice that your hands come closer together as you perform the positive phase of the rep. This adds an extra squeeze on your chest muscles and really improves the exercise. But suppose you feel *too much* pressure on your shoulder joints when you start or when you return to the starting position. In that case, adjust your range of motion in the exercise so that you don't stretch that far. It's better to do an exercise through a full range of motion—but not at the expense of injury. You can gradually improve your range of motion as your fitness improves. I should mention that there are also recumbent bench press machines. I find them less preferable, however, because of above-the-neck vascular congestion that can occur during their use.

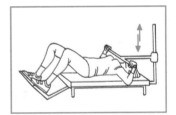

THE SEATED SHOULDER PRESS MACHINE

This machine exercises the muscles of your shoulders, your upper back, and your triceps. Again, be sure to keep your rear end back on the seat and your back firmly supported by the backrest. The height of the seat should be adjusted so that the handle grips are at or just above the level of the shoulders. As you raise the handles to perform the positive phase of each rep, be careful to avoid sliding forward or leaning forward—to avoid jerking your back. When you extend your arms upward, you might feel

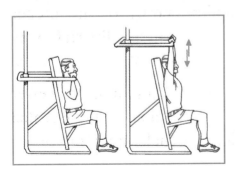

some discomfort in your shoulders or elbows. If that occurs, decrease the extension of your arms to a point just short of that. The same is true on the return to the starting position—shorten the return to a point where little or no discomfort is felt in your elbows and shoulders. Again, while it's better to perform the exercise through a complete range of motion, it's not worth the risk of injury. You can gradually increase your range of motion over a period of time with each exercise. The stretching exercises we've discussed can also be quite effective.

TRICEPS MACHINE EXERCISES

There are several different ways to exercise the triceps, the muscles in the back of your upper arm. If you've pre-fatigued your triceps with the seated bench press or vertical shoulder

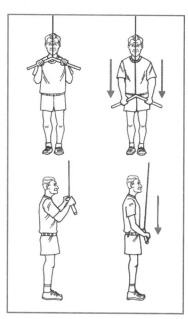

press, now is a good time to do your triceps. One technique is using the upper pulley attached to a triangular shaped bar. To assume your starting position, you should grasp the handles, keep your elbows tucked into your sides, and keep the point of the triangular bar just below your chin. Now slowly extend your arms downward to do the positive phase of the rep. To complete the rep, hold it for a count of one and then slowly return to the starting position.

In this exercise it's important to remember to keep your back straight and do *not* let the point of the triangular bar rise above the height of your chin. Also, don't bend your back and use your upper body weight to push the resistance downward. Avoid this by fixing your feet about 10 to 12 inches apart, or put one in

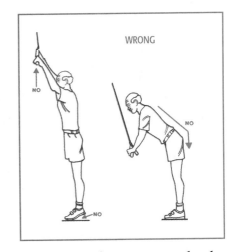

front of the other while keeping your elbows close to your body, slightly bending your knees, and tightening your abdominal muscles, while concentrating on keeping your back straight. The slight bend in your knees can help avoid any strain on your back, but you have to fix that position. In other words, don't bend and straighten your knees while doing the exercise, or you'll be using your body weight to move the resistance. Also, make sure the triangular bar has good grips or flanges, and wear exercise gloves so that the bar doesn't slip out of your hands and pop you in the chin!

Variations of this exercise movement can be done using a straight bar or rope, which will change the position of your hands. In this way, greater emphasis is placed on one or the other of the three parts of the muscle. Try to do these triceps exercises slowly, using light resistance. This will help you concentrate on tightening the triceps muscles and avoid compromising your form.

Some other very good triceps exercises are the seated arm extension apparatus and the dip machine. Don't forget that variation between machines can fend off muscle boredom and 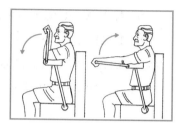 enhance your overall muscular fitness. There are also excellent floor exercises for the triceps, and some triceps exercises that can be done with dumbbells—but we'll discuss those in the next chapter.

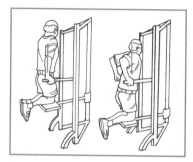

THE UPPER-BACK MACHINE

The upper-back machine exercises your mid- and upper-back muscles, shoulders, and arms. A side note: Since these back muscles are big, exercising them can burn a lot of calories!

Position yourself so that you're facing the machine and your chest is firmly placed against the padded support. The height of the seat should be adjusted so that the handles are just below the level of your shoulders. This pulling exercise is performed by 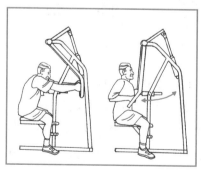 extending your arms, grasping the handles, and pulling against the resistance—toward yourself. The padded chest plate is used for support. To do this correctly, you must be seated with your chest firmly pressed against the chest support. If you're coming away from the chest support or off of the seat, you're doing it incorrectly. By using your legs, you're straining your low back—and you don't want to do that.

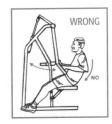

THE LAT PULL DOWN

The lat bar or upper pull-down machine is another pulling exercise for your upper back, shoulders, and arms. The positive phase of the rep involves pulling the bar down to a point level with your upper chest. The negative phase entails returning the bar to the starting position. You can use this machine instead of the upper-back machine or alternate between the two. If you use a wide grip on the lat bar and do the pull-down exercise behind your neck and across the back of your shoulders, you will be exercising your lower lat muscles.

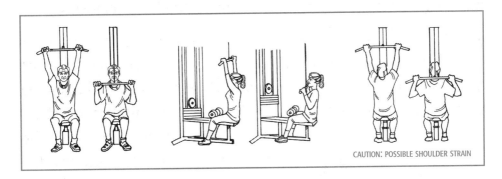

CAUTION: POSSIBLE SHOULDER STRAIN

"Lats" are the big muscles in the back that give the torsos of bodybuilders that "V" shape. They're actually called the *latissimus dorsi* muscles, but lats for short. Using the lat pull-down bar behind your back can really work out and build your lats. But that's not of interest for most of us. While some trainers encourage using a wide grip and doing the pull down behind your back, I'm a little concerned about that. It puts a lot of strain on the shoulder joints—and many of us aren't flexible enough to do this without getting hurt. You can get a very good workout by using a closer grip and doing the pull-downs in front of your chest. A variation is to do alternating sets with your palms facing forward, then with your palms facing backward. You can get a great workout of your upper back, shoulders, and arms this way.

There are a few additional tips I'd like to share with you: Adjust the height of the seat so there's a very slight bend in your elbows when you grip the bar. Whether your palms are facing forward or backward, grip the bar so there are about 10 to 12 inches between your hands. This is a good starting position for this exercise. You can vary this with closer or wider grips as you become accustomed to the exercise. When you pull down to do the positive phase of the rep, keep your feet flat and don't come off the seat.

Also, stay seated during the negative phase when you're returning to the starting position. People have a tendency to jerk themselves off the seat in this exercise. When they do this in the

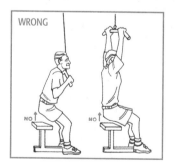

positive phase, they're using their body weight to get the resistance moving— and if they do it in the negative phase, they're also reducing the effectiveness of the exercise. Some of these machines have a padded support bar that goes across the top of your knees. This can keep you from rising up during the exercise. As always, do the exercise slowly. And make sure your grip is firm. It's a good idea to use exercise gloves so the bar doesn't slip from your sweaty hands.

Here's a variation of this machine that I prefer over the lat bar: It's a pull-down machine that has the handle grips set at a comfortable angle to reduce strain on the shoulder and elbow joints.

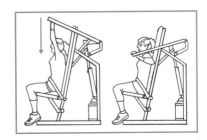

ARM CURL MACHINE

Now that you've pre-fatigued your arms with the upper-back machine or the lat pull machine, let's go over to the arm curl machine. This machine is designed to exercise the muscles in the front of your upper arms—such as your biceps. But it can also improve your grip and forearm muscles. It's very important that you adjust the seat so the backs of your upper arms rest comfortably on the padded supports. When you grip the handles, there should be a slight bend in your elbows, and the padded chest support should be flush against your torso. Keep it that way throughout the exercise. This will prevent you from coming off your seat and leaning forward during the

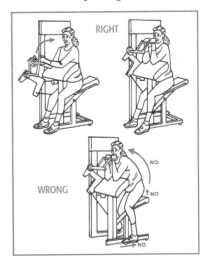

exercise. If you do, you will be using your back and your legs to help you move the resistance instead of your biceps—so sit tight.

The positive phase of the rep consists of flexing your arms against the resistance, and the negative phase consists of returning to the starting position. No other part of your body should change position. If you use an underhand grip, this exercise should concentrate its effort on the biceps. If you use an overhand grip, you exercise some of the other muscles in your arm such as the *brachialis* muscle. Do these arm curls slowly—to the count of four—and hold for the count of one. Sit tight and concentrate on good breathing. There are also some really great arm exercises you can do with dumbbells—but we'll get to that later.

THE SEATED LEG PRESS

The muscles in the thighs and legs are huge and strong. Exercising them can burn a lot of calories, increase the mineral density of our bones, and make us stronger, too. All of this adds up to better balance, greater endurance, and a decrease in falls and fractures. But be aware that these exercises put strain on the knee and hip joints. *If you've had orthopedic problems or surgery in these areas, it's important to check with your doctor to make sure these exercises would be appropriate for you.*

The classic exercise weightlifters use to build strong legs is known as "squats." We've all seen a weightlifter doing deep knee bends with a weight-loaded barbell across his or her shoulders. That's a squat. It's a great exercise for building huge, strong thighs, but it puts an enormous amount of strain on the knee joints, back, and shoulders. The deeper the squat the better the exercise—but also the greater risk of injury. That's why I think most people are better served by using the seated leg press machine. Why? We can isolate the exercise to these leg muscles alone and thus reduce the risk of injury.

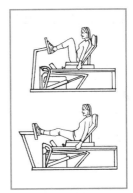

Bending your legs more than 90 degrees in this exercise puts additional stress on the ligaments of the knee and adds little to the desired benefits. In using the seated leg press machine, it's important to be seated so that your rear end is back on the seat, your knees bent, and your feet flat and placed firmly on the resistance pedals. Your toes should be pointing straight and your head bent forward. This is the starting position. The positive phase of each rep is performed by straightening your legs against the resistance. The negative phase is performed by returning to the starting position.

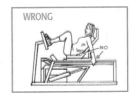

If you slide forward, you might strain your back. So keep your head bent forward; that can reduce strain on your back and also helps you maintain the proper form.

Remember, the deeper you flex those thighs, the better the exercise—but the greater the chance of injuring your knee or hip joints. Use a comfortable range of motion, and don't increase the resistance too quickly. You can increase your leg strength without exceeding your comfort zone. How? By gradually increasing the number of reps, sets, and resistance and then slowly increasing the degree of flexion as your comfort level permits. As always, there's no rush. Remember our motto: *Strain a little, gain a lot.*

To further strengthen your thigh muscles, slightly alter the position of your feet for a few reps or sets. If you point your toes slightly inward, you will put a little more strain on the muscles of your outer thigh. If you point your toes outward, you will give more exercise to the muscles of your inner thigh. Doing a few reps or sets this way can help to round out the development of your thigh muscles.

You can also exercise and strengthen your calf muscles with the seated leg press machine. As you know, the leg press is done with your feet flat on the resistance pedals. Keeping the balls and heels of your feet flush with the resistance pedals helps to incorporate the muscles in both the front (the quadriceps) and back (the hamstrings) of your thigh. But if you push the resistance with the balls of your feet, raising your heels up and off the pedals for a few reps or sets, you will also exercise your calf muscles.

You can further isolate the exercise to the calf muscles as follows: With your legs straight, push against the resistance with the balls of your feet. This moves the resistance away from your heels, allowing them to rise up from the pedals. Do this slowly, and then slowly return your heels to the resistance pedals. As you repeat this maneuver, you will feel your calf muscles getting pumped up.

THE SEATED LEG EXTENSION

The seated leg extension focuses on the muscles in the front of the thigh (the quadriceps). These muscles may have been pre-fatigued by exercising on the seated leg press. If so, this will decrease the amount of resistance, sets, or reps required to complete working them out. Note the seat and a shin pad on this machine—both of which can be adjusted to your size and the length of your legs. Sitting on the machine with your knees bent over the seat and your feet behind the shin pad is the starting position. Be sure to sit back on the seat with your back flush against the support.

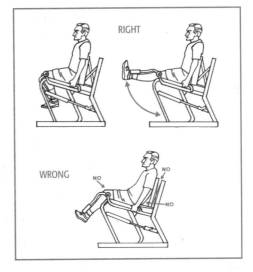

There is a handle on each side of the seat that you can grasp to stabilize and secure your position. If you're using Keiser equipment, there's a button on each of these handles that will allow you to easily increase or decrease the resistance for the exercise. The positive phase of the rep consists of slowly straightening the legs against the resistance and holding for a count of one. The negative phase consists of slowly returning to the starting position. It's very important not to slide forward on the seat. If you do, you'll be straining your lower back. This is a fabulous exercise for strengthening and defining the quadriceps. You can get even better definition of these muscles by concentrating on the muscle contraction as you straighten your legs and holding them out there for a count of three or four between the positive and negative phase of the reps.

THE SEATED LEG CURL

The seated leg curl is a fabulous exercise for the muscles in the back of your thigh (hamstrings). These muscles play an important role in walking, running, stair climbing, and maintaining balance. Most leg exercises work out the quadriceps—the muscles in the front of the thighs. That's why our 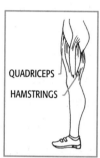 quadriceps muscles get much stronger than our hamstrings. For better balance, our hamstrings should be about two-thirds as strong as our quadriceps—but in most of us, they're not even close. This imbalance in strength, together with a failure to do proper stretching, is responsible for many falls and injuries. I'm sure that many of you have heard of professional athletes who were sidelined because of a *pulled hamstring*.

Note that this machine has two padded plates. Place your knees above the padded plate closest to you and your feet on top of the extended plate. The seat and other parts of the machine 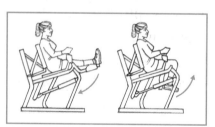 can be adjusted to accommodate your size. Sit back on the seat with your legs extended and a slight bend at your knees. Your back should be flush against the back support. Keep a firm grip on the handles to help fix your position. This is the starting position for this exercise.

The positive phase of the rep is performed as you bend and slowly curl your legs backward. Hold it there for a count of two or three. The negative phase is performed as you return to the starting position. Here again, the exercise should be done slowly and with perfect form. Try to do three sets of eight reps with a one-minute rest between sets. There are a number of different machines to exercise hamstrings besides this one. I like the seated variety because it offers more protection against back strain. But whatever hamstring exercises you do, *please—don't forget to stretch these muscles when you're done.*

THE ABDOMINAL MUSCLES

Now let's talk about exercising our abdominal muscles, or what are commonly referred to as our "abs." A lot of people don't realize the importance of these muscles. They think this kind of exercise is only for the purpose of producing a sexy-looking washboard or sixpack appearance to their belly. Not so! The abs assist you in respiration, in facilitating bowel evacuations, and, of equal importance, in maintaining the integrity of your low back. Weak abs not only predispose you to developing hernias, they let your potbelly protrude so that it pulls on your low back. On the other hand, well-conditioned and strong abs counterbalance your stronger back muscles, producing greater stability in your lower back. Conditioning your abdominal muscles is one of the best and most effective ways of preventing or alleviating lower-back problems. You'll be amazed at how much better you and your back feel when you strengthen these muscles! While less important, a marvelous side benefit can be a slimmer and more attractive appearance.

THE ABDOMINAL CRUNCH MACHINE

Floor exercises to strengthen the abdominal muscles are among my favorites (more about them in the next chapter), but the abdominal crunch machine can also give you a magnificent workout. This machine can be used as an alternative or in addition to floor exercises—and it's particularly useful for people who have difficulty getting down to or rising up from the floor.

Starting position: Sit on the machine facing the padded chest support. Be sure to adjust the seat so the upper level of the chest support is at the same level as your upper chest. Your feet should be flat on the floor and comfortably but firmly positioned behind the stationary foot supports. Place your hands and arms firmly on the handles.

The positive phase of each rep consists of bending forward and squeezing and crunching the abdominal muscles into contraction.

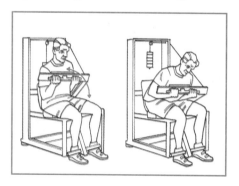

The negative phase consists of returning to the starting position. Do both phases of this exercise slowly, and squeeze the contraction between the positive and negative phase for a count of three or four.

Some of us will do better with three sets of 8 to 15 or more reps using light resistance, and others will feel they've gotten a better workout with fewer reps and more resistance. *If you've had hip surgery, check with your doctor before doing this exercise.*

VERY SLOW RESISTANCE TRAINING

Some experts have recommended still slower repetitions—perhaps a 14-second rep, seven seconds in the active direction and seven in the return phase of the exercise. This kind of program usually involves doing only one set of five reps of each movement once a week as a total workout. There is some evidence that this approach can significantly increase muscle mass. The downside is that it requires much concentration and may encourage breath holding. Advocates claim it is safer and more effective. While this may work for some folks, I think the jury is still out on these issues—and I have very serious concerns about the health benefits of exercising only once a week.

CONCENTRIC AND ECCENTRIC MUSCLE CONTRACTION

Generally speaking, I am an advocate of doing resistance training with slow reps. Why? Because it decreases the chance of muscle injury and increases the rate of muscle development. When you are lifting weight, your muscle is contracting and shortening. This is *concentric muscle contraction.* When you are slowly lowering the weight, your muscle is contracted against resistance as it is lengthening. This is called *eccentric muscle contraction.* Since you can lower more weight than you can lift, you might improve your muscle mass and bone strength even more effectively by prolonging the return phase of each rep. So if you feel you have to decrease the time of the positive phase of your reps (concentric contraction), try to prolong the return phase (eccentric contraction). For example, you might do your reps with a two-second positive phase and a six- or seven-second return phase.

FAST-TWITCH FIBERS

It's important to note that there are basically two kinds of muscle fibers in your muscles: white muscle fibers (fast-twitch fibers) and red muscle fibers (slow-twitch fibers). Many experts believe that the fast-twitch fibers are more important in establishing quick reflexes, maintaining proprioception (awareness of your body's position and orientation), and generating quick power surges. After you've achieved a modicum of fitness, you might get the best of both worlds by doing the last one or two reps of each set very slowly (stimulating the red fibers) and then stimulating the white fibers by doing a set of reps as fast as you can—but with half of the resistance you normally use so as to avoid possible injury.

WHOLE-BODY VIBRATION (WBV)

Recent studies have shown that the appropriate application of whole-body vibration (WBV) has many benefits. It can improve bone density, produce stretch reflexes in muscle spindles to enhance muscle conditioning, improve flexibility, increase the release of human growth hormone, and decrease the production of cortisol. While there are several devices on the market, the Power Plate used at Nifty after Fifty centers can be adjusted to produce 30 to 50 stretch reflexes a second. The magnitude of the stretch can be adjusted to vary from 2–4 mm to as much as 4–6 mm. You can gradually build up to a 10-minute workout on the Power Plate—believed by many to be the equivalent of a 45-minute, moderate strength-training session. You can exercise and burn calories simply by standing on the machine or perhaps enhance your workout by doing selected movements and exercises while vibrating. Contraindications to the use of this device are few (joint replacements, orthopedic screws, pacemakers, etc.), but before using WBV, review any such conditions with an informed trainer. At Nifty after Fifty we've found the Power Plate to be a great 30- to 60-second warm-up and cool-down machine—possibly by enhancing the production and release of neurotransmitters.

LOOKING BACK, LOOKING FORWARD

CHAPTER 13 REVIEW ...

♦ In only eight weeks of resistance training, you can realize an amazing increase in muscle strength.

♦ State-of-the-art conditioning can best be achieved through the use of resistance training machines that decrease the effects of inertia.

♦ The ABCs of strength training are A: perfect form, B: proper breathing technique, and C: gradual progression.

♦ For maximum effectiveness, training sessions should be scheduled several times a week and always preceded and followed by stretching exercises.

CHAPTER 14 PREVIEW ...

♦ Is it possible to maintain an effective exercise program at home if I can't make it to a gym?

♦ Why is it important to exercise different muscle groups on different days?

♦ What modifications must I make in order to do push-ups and sit-ups safely?

♦ What special exercises can help to correct balance problems? How can I incorporate these simple exercises into my normal daily activities?

14

SIT DOWN AND SHAPE UP:
Strength and Balance Exercises You Can Do at Home

An active mind cannot exist in an inactive body.
—General George S. Patton

*Today, the most common form
of physical abuse is disuse.*
—Stephen Seiler

I know there are many reasons why some of us simply can't get to the gym on a regular basis. Others, after learning how to train in the gym, might prefer to continue strength and balance training at home. Perhaps some of you might even want to set up a gym at home. Many manufacturers produce excellent strength-training equipment (Keiser, Cybex, Bowflex, etc.) that can be used to furnish a home gym. Also, there are a variety of treadmills and stationary bikes on the market you can use for cardiopulmonary conditioning.

That said, excellent strength training, balance training, and endurance exercises can also be done at home without a lot of fancy equipment. Some of the strength and balance exercises are so important that we should all practice them, regardless of where we work out—at home or in the gym. The equipment you need is very little: a chair, a floor, and a couple of pairs of dumbbells and ankle weights. You can also make do by using half-gallon plastic containers with handles. By filling them with varying amounts of water or sand, you can change the weight resistance for different exercises and use them as you would dumbbells. Alternatively, bags of sand can be used like dumbbells. Ankle weights, which can be bought in almost any sporting goods store, would also be beneficial—but they're not essential.

PRINCIPLES

The principles and precautions of resistance training are the same whether you're at home or in the gym. Because they're so very important, let's do a quick review: You will want to do a set of 8 to 15 repetitions (reps) of each movement with perfect form. You should gradually work toward doing two or three sets of each exercise and, as you progress, shortening the rest period between sets. Start slowly at first, using minimal resistance. When you find you can easily do three sets of an exercise, increase the number of reps in each set to 10 and then to 12 or 15. When you can do two or three sets of 12 to 15 reps in each set, you're ready to advance. Slightly increase the weight or resistance and go back to eight reps in each set. Continuing this progressive process will challenge your muscles and make them stronger. It will also increase your endurance for repetitive motion. Some of us may not be able to do eight reps of one or more of the exercises. Well, so be it. Remember the old Chinese saying: *Every journey begins by taking the first step.* If you can't do eight reps, do one or two or three reps. The point is to *gradually* try to increase your ability. If you try—and if you stay with it—you will improve.

Take a deep breath at the starting position of each repetition and breathe out against the resistance. Then, fill your lungs with air during the return to the starting position. Repeat this sequence of inhaling and exhaling with each rep. Between sets, stretch the muscles you've exercised before going on to the next kind of movement. *And, first and foremost—do your stretching exercises every day, even on days that you don't do resistance or endurance training.*

FREQUENCY

Bear in mind that exercise stimulates all of the magnificent biological mechanisms that make your muscles grow and become stronger. Also remember that your muscles grow and increase in strength while they're resting, *not* while you're exercising them. So if you're going to strength-train everyday, alternate the muscle groups that you work out. For example: You can do your upper-body muscles on Monday, Wednesday, and Friday and your lower-body muscles on Tuesday, Thursday, and Saturday. If you're going to strength-train two or three days a week, then exercise both your upper- and lower-body muscles on the same days.

Recent studies suggest that if you increase the intensity and duration of your workout, most mature adults can probably do as well by strength-training twice a week. If you use this schedule, I suggest something like Tuesday and Friday strength-training sessions. This permits one 48-hour rest period and one 72-hour rest period between resistance exercise sessions. For some of us, this added period of rest is beneficial to muscle growth and strength. It also allows more time for endurance training on the other days.

CHAIR STAND

Let's start with the lower body. Leg strength, after all, is extremely important in maintaining balance and preventing falls—so all the muscles in our legs play an important role. The chair stand exercise involves most of these muscles, so it's one of the most important exercises.

Begin by placing a pillow behind the small of the back for some support. Sit up straight with your arms crossed over your chest. Then stand up straight without leaning the shoulders forward—and do this slowly to the count of three. Then, sit back down—again, slowly to the count of three. That's what I mean when I say, "*Sit down to shape up and repeat and repeat and repeat.*" Do a set of 8 to 15 reps, and then rest and do another set or two.

Some of us may have to use our hands to help us with this movement, and that's okay. The idea is to gradually improve

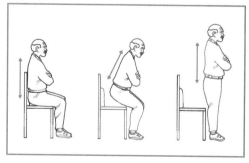

our performance in doing this exercise so that we don't have to use our hands at all. But, whether using your hands or not, keep your back straight and avoid jerking motions.

You'll find this exercise more difficult to perform if you use a chair that has a low seat, so start with a chair that has a high seat. (Switch to a chair with a lower seat when the exercise becomes easy.) If your chair is too low for you at the start, raise the height of the seat by adding a firm cushion. When and if this exercise becomes too easy for you, you can increase the resistance by performing the same exercise while holding dumbbells or a telephone book.

KNEE EXTENSION AND DORSI-FLEXION OF THE FOOT

This movement will strengthen the muscles in the front of the thigh known as the *quadriceps*. It also develops the muscles of your shin—in the front of your lower leg. To strengthen your quadriceps, begin by sitting in the chair with your feet hanging freely or allowing only the balls of your feet or your toes to touch the floor. You can do this by sitting up straight and placing some rolled up towels on the chair under your knees, or you could also raise the seat with a firm cushion.

Once comfortably seated, support yourself by placing your hands on the sides of the seat near the front. Now, extend one leg slowly to the count of three seconds and hold it out there while flexing and squeezing your foot and your toes toward you. Then lower your leg back to the starting position—slowly to the count of three seconds. Do two or three sets of 8 to 12 reps each—first with one leg, then with the other. As your confidence increases, you

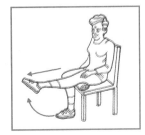

might be able to do both legs at one time. And as your strength further increases, it will be time to buy some ankle weights.

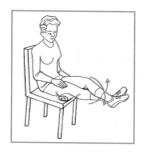 You might vary this exercise by crossing your feet and squeezing your thighs together when your legs are extended—making a "scissors" movement. This will also help to exercise some of the muscles of your inner thighs.

What's the reason for flexing the foot upward during the hold part of the movement? It's to help strengthen the muscles of your shin—the front of your lower leg. These muscles are referred to as the dorsi-flexors of the foot because their function is to flex the foot upward. When those muscles are weak, your step gets sloppy; your toes and the ball of your foot tend to drag when you bring your foot forward. This can increase the tendency to shuffle, stumble, and trip.

These muscles not only help you walk, but they also help you climb stairs and take your foot off the gas pedal to place it on the brake. So when you have your knee extended and your foot flexed upward toward you, squeeze those muscles in the front of your shin—the dorsi-flexors of the foot. Few people think to exercise these muscles. But they're more important than most people realize in maintaining balance and agility and avoiding tripping. As an added benefit, this movement also helps to stretch the muscles in the back of your calf.

Another way to work the front of your lower leg is to sit on the chair with your feet flat on the floor. Keep your heels on the floor as you raise the balls of your feet upward (off the floor) and curl your toes toward your head. Hold it there and squeeze for three seconds. When that 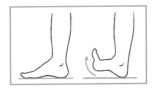 becomes too easy for you, you can hold telephone books or dumbbells on your knees to add resistance.

CALF MUSCLE AND ANKLE MUSCLE EXERCISES

To work your calf muscles on the back of your lower leg, support yourself by holding on to the back of a chair with your 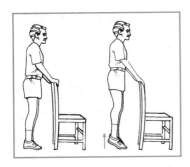 feet flat on the floor. Then, to the slow count of three, raise up on the balls of your feet—on to your tippy, tippy toes—then hold it for one second. Next, slowly lower yourself back to the starting position— 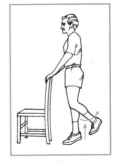 also to the count of three seconds. Do two or three sets of about 8 to 15 reps in each set. This exercise will strengthen the muscles of your calf and your ankle. When it gets easy, try it with one leg at a time.

KNEE FLEXION EXERCISE FOR THE BACK OF YOUR THIGH

The next exercise will strengthen the muscles in the back of your thigh—your hamstring muscles. Using the same position and supporting yourself by holding on to the back of the chair,

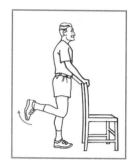

bend one leg backward and then upward at the knee so that the heel of your foot comes as close to the back of your thigh as possible. Again, do this slowly to the count of three or four seconds and hold it there for a second. Then slowly return to the starting position to the count of three or four seconds. Do two or three sets of 8 to 15 reps with each leg. Alternate your legs for each set. When this gets to be easy, add ankle weights.

HIP MUSCLE EXERCISES

The next three movements will strengthen the muscles that surround the hip and the upper thigh. Here again, ankle weights would be very helpful, particularly as these exercises become too easy for you.

Hip flexion

Strengthening the muscles that flex your hips is a good way to prevent shuffling and falls. While many gyms have excellent machines for this exercise, you can easily do it at home. As you progress, ankle weights can be added to further build your strength. While standing off to the side of the chair and using the back of the chair for support, bend your leg upward, moving your knee toward your abdomen as far as you can. It's important that you stand straight—don't bend your back. Do this slowly to the count of three or four seconds and hold it for a second

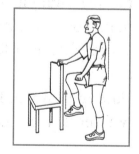

before slowly returning to the starting position. With each leg do one set of 8 to 15 reps, and then try another one or two sets.

Side leg raise

The side leg raise strengthens the muscles on your outer thigh and hip. Stand directly behind a chair and support yourself by holding the back of the chair. Keep your back and your legs straight as you raise one leg outward toward the side about 6 to 12 inches. Do this slowly to the count of three or four seconds and hold it out there for a count of one second. Then, slowly return to the starting position. Do one set of 8 to 15 reps with each leg, and then do another one or two more sets.

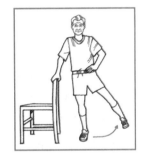

Hip extension

The hip extension exercise will strengthen the muscles of your buttocks and your lower back. Stand a foot (or a little more) behind a chair with your feet about 6 to 12 inches apart. Support yourself by placing your hands on the back of the chair. Bend slightly forward at the hips—*not at the waist*. This is the starting position for this movement. Raise one leg straight back, keeping the leg straight. Don't bend your knee or point your toes. Raise your leg slowly to the count of three or four seconds and hold it for a second before slowly returning to the starting position. Do one set of 8 to 15 reps with each leg, and then repeat one or two more sets.

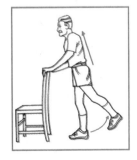

UPPER-BODY STRENGTH TRAINING AT HOME
STRENGTHENING THE MUSCLES OF THE SHOULDER GIRDLE

This next set of exercises consists of three movements aimed at strengthening the muscles of the shoulder girdle. They are best performed with dumbbells, but as suggested earlier, half-gallon plastic jugs or bags of sand can be used as substitutes. Please note: Your position in the chair is very important. Sit in the chair with your back straight and your feet flat on the floor. Spread your feet so that they are about as far apart as your shoulders, and hold a dumbbell in each hand. Now you're ready to start the first movement.

With each of these exercises, start with a weight that is light enough for you to do 8 to 15 reps in each set with perfect form. When you can do two or three sets of 12 to 15 reps, increase the weight slightly. As you get stronger you can gradually continue to increase the weight—but not until you can do two or three sets of 12 to 15 reps.

Side arm-raise

This exercise will strengthen the muscles of the side of your shoulder girdle. With a dumbbell in each hand, your palms facing inward and your arms bent slightly at the elbows, slowly raise

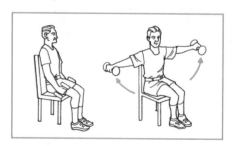

your arms upward on each side until they are at about the level of your shoulders. Do this lift to the count of two, hold it for a second, and then slowly return to the starting position.

Forward arm-raise

This exercise will strengthen the muscles of the front of the shoulder girdle. Start with your arms down at your sides and your palms facing backward. Then raise both arms upward to shoulder height. Do this slowly to the count of two seconds, and hold it for a second before slowly returning to the starting position.

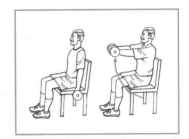

Vertical rows

The vertical row movement is a fabulous exercise to strengthen the muscles of your upper back (the trapezius muscles), your neck muscles, and the muscles of your shoulder girdle. This exercise will also help to strengthen and pre-fatigue the muscles of the front of your arms in preparation for the next group of exercises to be discussed (curls). Vertical rows can be done standing or sitting. Here's how: With a dumbbell in each hand and your palms facing backward, pull the dumbbells straight up to the level of your upper chest so that your elbows are pointing out. Do this slowly, without jerking your arms or your back. Hold it for a second or two, and then slowly lower your hands back to the starting position. Try one to three sets of 8 to 12 reps.

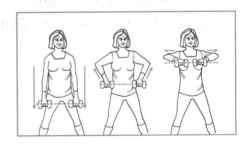

Backward arm-raise

This exercise, which strengthens the muscles of the back of your shoulder girdle, involves a slight change in position. Put your feet close together and bend forward at the hips (not at the waist). Make sure the dumbbells you're holding are alongside your feet. This is the starting position for this movement. Now slowly raise your arms upward and outward—like a bird

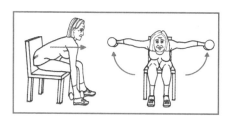

spreading its wings—to shoulder level to the count of three or four seconds. Hold it there for a second before slowly returning to the starting position.

ARM CURLS

This next series of movements, which can be done in the sitting or standing position, will strengthen the muscles in the front of your upper arms as well as your forearms. Try to do one to three sets of eight reps for each of the following exercises. When you're able to do eight reps of each exercise easily, try to increase the number of reps in each set to 10 or even 12 or 15. Then add more weight and start again with eight reps and so on. *It's very important that you pay strict attention to form and avoid swinging the dumbbells.* Now, for the first exercise:

Twist curls

With your palms facing inward and a dumbbell in each hand, slowly bend your arms upward at the elbow. As you do this, turn your hands so that your palms point toward the front of your shoulders. Proceed as you have with the other exercises demonstrated, doing this movement slowly to the count of three or four seconds and holding for one second. Then slowly return to the starting position. *A very important aspect of the arm curl* 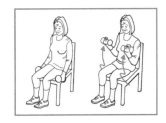 exercises is to keep your elbows firmly tucked into your sides during the entire movement. Don't lean forward, and don't jerk the weight upward.* If you do, you'll be using your back and your shoulder muscles to raise the weight instead of isolating the exercise to the arm muscles—you won't get the full benefit of the exercise. Also, be careful not to swing the weights to get the movement going. Doing curls by swinging the weights and using your back to raise the weight are called *cheat curls*. This is less likely to happen if you do the exercise while sitting.

If you do the exercise in the standing position, however, bend your knees slightly to take strain off your back. You can also decrease the potential for straining your back by placing one foot in front of the other. When you have finished a set of 8 to 10 reps of the twist curls, rest for a couple of minutes before doing another one or two sets.

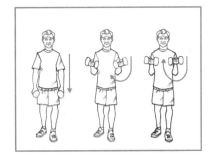

Traditional curls

If you really want to develop sharp-looking biceps, you can try a set or two of *traditional curls*. Start with the dumbbells at your side and the palms of your hands facing forward. There's no twisting in this movement. With your hands at your sides and your palms facing forward, flex your elbows upward so that your palms are facing the front of your shoulders.

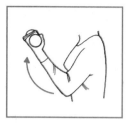

Remember to keep your elbows tucked closely against your body throughout this movement. Do the movement slowly to the count of three seconds, and hold it for a second while concentrating on the squeeze. Then slowly return to the starting position. Do 8 to 12 repetitions, and then rest for two minutes. Do another set or two, and then try one to three sets of reverse curls.

Reverse curls

This is basically the same movement, but done with your palms facing backward. Bend your arms upward at the elbow so that the backs of your hands are facing the front of your

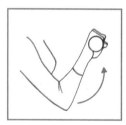

shoulders. Again, make the movement slowly and then slowly return to the starting position. Try to do 8 to 10 reps before resting for about two minutes. Then try another set or two if you like.

EXERCISES FOR THE BACK OF THE ARM

The next set of exercises are designed to strengthen the back of your upper arms (the triceps muscles). While there are several very good exercises you can do at home to strengthen these muscles, one that involves dumbbells is called the "triceps extension." Let's start with that.

Triceps extension

Position yourself slightly toward the front of the chair seat with your feet about one foot apart. Hold the dumbbell in one hand with your palm facing inward, and bend your arm so that the weight hangs over and behind your shoulder. Immobilize and support the upper part of this arm with your other hand. This is the starting position.

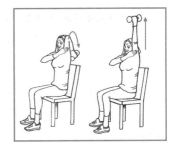

Now slowly lift the weight straight up toward the ceiling to the count of three, and then slowly return to the starting position. Keep your back straight throughout the movement, and concentrate on keeping the upper part of your arm immobilized. Do a set of 8 to 15 reps before doing a set with the other arm. Now take a one- or two-minute rest and repeat the exercise with each arm one or two more times.

Shoulder press

The shoulder press is another good exercise for your triceps and also helps to strengthen the muscles of the shoulder girdle. Here's how to do it: Hoist the dumbbells to shoulder height and hold them there with your palms facing inward toward your chest. This is the starting position for this movement. Now, straighten your arms by slowly lifting the dumbbells straight up over your head. As you lift the dumbbells, rotate your hands so that your palms are facing forward. Then

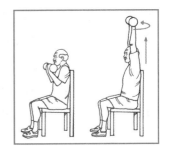

slowly return to the starting position. Again, do about 8 to 15 reps before resting for a minute or two. Then try another one or two sets. Alternatively, you can do one arm at a time, or alternate arms.

The chair dip

This exercise strengthens the triceps as well as some of your chest and shoulder muscles. You need a chair with sturdy armrests. When you sit in the chair, the armrests should be slightly higher than your waist. If the armrests are too high, using cushions to sit higher can usually help. (If they're too low, however, you probably need to use a different chair.)

Place your hands on the armrests, just slightly toward the front of your waist, and lean forward a little. Keep your back straight and lift yourself off the seat by straightening your arms. Do

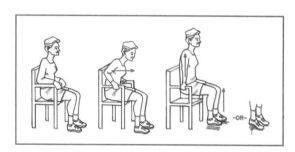

this to the slow count of three and hold it for the count of one. Then slowly lower yourself onto the seat. Try to do 8 to 12 reps before resting for a minute or two. Then try to do another set or two. Many of you may not have the strength to do this exercise without using your legs to help you—and that's okay. Over time, as your strength increases, you can try to use your legs less and less until you may not need to use them at all.

Push-ups

Push-ups are among the most popular floor exercises used to strengthen the muscles in the back of the arms (the triceps) and also the chest muscles. These can be very hard for some of us who haven't exercised for a long time—but with modifications, this exercise can be useful to many of us. Let's first demonstrate the classical push-up before introducing the modifications.

The classic push-up is done off the floor with the hands placed at shoulder level. The chest is slowly lowered to the floor and then raised to the starting position.

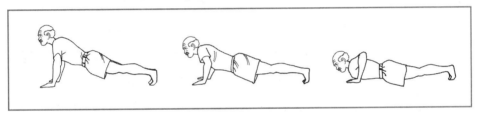

By varying the position of the hands—by placing them farther apart, closer together, or higher than shoulder level—emphasis can be placed on different aspects of the musculature of the arms and shoulder girdle. (Some athletes do push-ups on their fingertips, and some even do one-handed push-ups!)

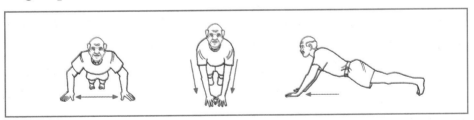

All fours modified floor push-ups

Many of us who can't do regular push-ups will be able to do a modified push-up by positioning ourselves on all fours (on our hands and knees). Place your hands on the floor slightly in front of your shoulders and about as wide apart as your shoulders.

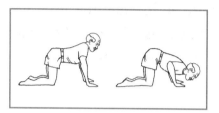

This is the starting position for this exercise. Lower your chest slowly to the floor and then use your arms to lift your shoulders back to the starting position.

You can vary this position by putting your hands directly under your shoulders and moving your knees back three to six inches. As your strength improves you can continue to vary the

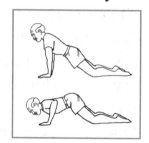

position of your hands and knees. You might then be able to increase the number of repetitions and possibly progress to full floor push-ups. But if doing push-ups from the all-fours position is too strenuous for you, you might try wall push-ups.

Wall push-ups

Doing push-ups against the wall is a modification that most all of us will be able to do. Stand at arms-length from the wall.

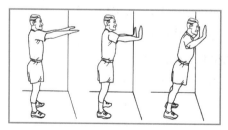

Position yourself so that your fingertips can just about touch the wall. With your back and your arms straight, lean forward so that the palms of your hands are flush with the wall. Support yourself there with straight arms and a straight back. This is the starting position for this movement. Now slowly bend your arms so that your face and upper chest become almost flush with the wall. Then slowly return to the starting position. Do a set of three, five, or as many as you can, up to 15 reps. Rest for about a minute and repeat the exercise. Then gradually increase the number of reps. When it becomes easy, you can try the modified floor push-ups on all fours.

ABDOMINAL MUSCLE EXERCISES

The next exercises strengthen our abdominal muscles—and might even give us a good-looking sixpack. These muscles are extremely important to maintaining a healthy low back and abdomen. They're also important to breathing and to other normal daily living activities—such as the simple or sometimes not so simple act of having a bowel movement. We've already discussed the use of the abdominal crunch machines in the gym. Now we're going to show you how to exercise these muscles at home. The first kind of ab exercises we'll discuss are concentration exercises.

Concentration abs

Concentration abs can be done standing, sitting, or lying on your back. Let's try the standing one first. Stand with your back flush against the wall. Now, suck in your abdomen. Envision the front of your abdomen moving back toward your spine— squeeze it in for a second or two. Then relax before doing it again—a little harder. Then relax. Do two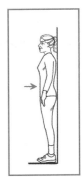

or three sets of 5 to 30 reps. Longer and harder squeezes can produce better results than quick, more numerous repetitions. You can do the same exercise while lying on your back or even sitting in a chair. What could be more convenient? In the chair, you can do concentration ab exercises at work or at a meeting or while watching TV. No one will even realize you're working out—as long as you control your facial expression!

Abdominal crunches

Let's move on now to abdominal crunches you can do on the floor. An exercise mat would be helpful, but not essential. A soft carpet and a towel are just as good.

The classic exercise for the abs is the sit-up. The starting position consists of lying flat on your back with your arms bent at the elbows and hands clasped behind your head. Note that the legs are stretched flat on the floor and the feet are spread

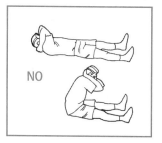

apart about 18 inches. The exercise is performed by sitting up and touching your elbows to your knees and then returning to the starting position. *Note: This is precisely the kind of exercise I want you to avoid.*

Doing this exercise with straight legs puts an enormous strain on your back. So the first lesson you must learn is *not to do this exercise with straight legs.* Always do sit-ups with bent knees and only with bent knees. This will take the strain off your back.

You can do sit-ups with your hands clasped behind your head or with your arms folded in front of you. You can also do them by coming only halfway up and squeezing or "crunching" your abdominal muscles.

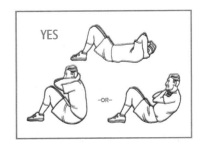

I have often observed people doing sit-ups as fast as they can in an effort to do more and more reps. But the actual number of reps is far less important than the strength of the muscular contraction. The important thing is not speed but *trying to squeeze or crunch your abs throughout the exercise.* Hold it for a second or two at the halfway point before slowly returning to the starting position. Do as many as you can. Then rest for a minute or two and try another set or two.

Some fitness trainers insist that this type of exercise should include a variation in which each elbow is alternatively made to touch the opposite knee. They believe that some of the muscles on the sides of our abdomen (known as the *oblique* muscles) are better exercised this way. While this seems to have merit, there is little scientific evidence to support this contention.

Sporting goods stores and other sales outlets have a number of different kinds of equipment especially designed to support your head and neck during these movements. Others focus on roller-wheel mechanisms that can exercise your abs and some of the other muscles of your trunk at the same time. These are interesting and novel approaches that can serve to introduce some variety to your workout.

DISTURBANCES IN BALANCE

As noted earlier, fractures are among the common causes of death in the elderly. Most often, these fractures are caused by falls associated with balance deficits. Among older adults, balance problems can result from a number of different conditions. To name a few common causes: disturbances in the inner ear, visual disturbances, vascular disease involving the circulation to the brain, medications, and muscle weakness. *Severe disturbances in balance—or even mild disturbances of recent onset—should be evaluated by your doctor.*

PRECAUTIONS AGAINST FALLING

The good news is that you can lower your risk of serious injury secondary to falls by following a few simple precautions.

- First and foremost, begin to strengthen the muscles of your lower extremities—and get going on a balance training program.

- To make your bones stronger, take the medications, vitamins, and supplements (calcium and vitamin D) recommended by your doctor.

- Ask your doctor or pharmacist to review your other medications to determine what, if any, role they might be playing in causing lightheadedness or drowsiness.

- Identify risky habits. For example, don't walk with your hands in your pockets. Why? If you lose your balance and start to fall, you might not be able to remove your hands fast enough to grab onto some support or break your fall.

◆ Improve the safety of your surroundings by wearing non-slip shoes and placing non-slip mats and handrails in the bath, the shower, and on staircases.

◆ Be certain that the lighting is adequate throughout your household. Also check that your carpeting is free of hazardous rumples.

◆ Some of us older folks notice marked dizziness with sudden changes in position. This is common with inner ear problems and also with sudden changes in blood pressure—sometimes secondary to one of our medications. If you've been lying down for a while, don't sit up too quickly. And beware of standing up suddenly after a long period of sitting. *If you suffer from this type of balance disturbance, it's important to take the time to stabilize when you change position.* If you're dizzy when you sit up from the reclining position, sit still for a moment and support yourself until you feel stable. Don't try to stand until you are. Then, when you stand, support yourself with one hand on a chair or a tabletop until you feel stable enough to walk. Don't start walking until you feel secure. These simple precautions might prevent a fall and spare you the grief of a major bone fracture.

BALANCE TRAINING

To strengthen your gait—and to some extent improve your balance—try walking in the shallow end of a swimming pool or taking classes in aquabatics. But the most effective device I've used to improve balance is the Functional Trainer made by

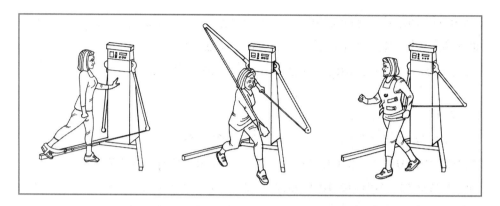

Keiser. At Nifty after Fifty, we've used this machine for many strength exercises, but its greatest application is in improving balance and strengthening gait. With the use of special vests and belts, air pressure resistance can be adjusted by a tenth of a pound at a time. Those who use it can gradually improve the strength of their forward, backward, and side-stepping gait— avoiding falls and fractures. While challenging and improving your balance, it also strengthens the core of your body. Several football teams use the Functional Trainer—particularly to train their linebackers. It has a significant advantage over the use of swimming pool aquabatics because the pressure can be regulated (increased or decreased), it avoids the false sense of security provided by the buoyancy of a pool, and it can be used with a walker or even with crutches or a cane.

The leg and hip exercises we've demonstrated for strength training are also extremely valuable in terms of improving balance. A stronger lower body, in and of itself, will improve your balance. If you are doing your strength training at home, you can integrate balance training into these movements. But even if you do most of your strength training in the gym, you should add these movements to your routine—purely for the purpose of enhancing your sense of equilibrium.

STRENGTH AND BALANCE

Let's revisit some of these movements, redirecting our focus from strength training to balance improvement. These movements include the side leg raise, the hip flexion, the hip extension, the calf muscle exercise, the dorsi-flexer foot exercises, and the chair stand. In most of these exercises we've stressed the importance of holding onto the back of a chair for support. But you can improve your balance even more if, as your strength improves, your reliance on the support gradually decreases. Example: In doing the side leg raise, try to gradually

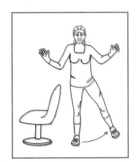

decrease your reliance on the chair for support—hold on with two fingertips, and when you feel more secure, try one fingertip. Hold the position for several seconds with each leg. As your balance improves, try letting go for a few seconds—LOOK, MA! NO HANDS!—as long as support is nearby. Then you might even try it with your eyes closed for a few seconds. Repeat this with the hip flexion and hip extension movements and the calf exercises (the toe stand).

EVERYDAY ACTIVITIES

Wherever you are in the course of your everyday activities, you can practice balance training—by standing on one foot for

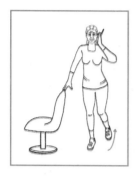

several seconds and then on the other foot. You can do this while talking on the phone or waiting in line at a store. When you rise from a chair, practice getting up without using your hands for assistance. The more frequently you try this, the better chance you give your balance to improve.

Heel-to-toe walk

You can try specific walking exercises to improve your balance. One of the best is the heel-to-toe walk. This is done by placing one foot progressively in front of the other, with the heel

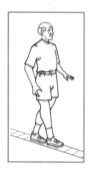

of one foot touching the toes of the other foot. This can be made even more difficult by envisioning an imaginary line about three to four inches wide. (A 10- to 20-foot length of toilet paper on a smooth, uncarpeted floor can be very useful here.) Try to do a heel-to-toe walk without breaking or disrupting the paper.

Eye exercises

Whether or not you can actually improve your vision with eye exercises is controversial. I believe, however, that there is real value to eye exercises that improve the motion of the eye. I also recommend some exercises that can help improve your focus and hand-eye coordination. Improved vision and eye-limb coordination can have a very positive effect on your balance. Clearly, there is no downside to doing these exercises. And even more importantly, they're not time-consuming. You can do them almost anytime and almost anywhere—but you have to take your glasses off! There are a number of variations to these exercises. Let's go over the three or four that I like the best.

◆ **Clock rotation:** Some research has shown that exercising the muscles that move the eyes (called the *extraocular* muscles) can improve vision. Better yet, the research also shows that the improvement is sometimes immediately noticeable. Imagine that you are looking at a *very large* clock. First, concentrate on the center of the clock, and then move your eyes up to the 12 o'clock position—as far up as you can. Hold them there for two or three seconds before returning your eyes to the center position on the clock. Now repeat the same movement to the one o'clock position and then to the two o'clock position and so on. After each hour, return to the starting position at the center of the imaginary clock. You can also try "eye rolls." Slowly roll and stretch your eyes as far as possible around the clock—from the one o'clock position through to the 12 o'clock position and then back again.

◆ **Far-to-near focus:** Did you know that straining to focus our eyes over years of reading, working at a computer, or other kinds of near-point focusing actually changes the shape of our eyes? Over time, our eyes become rounder and fatter—partly as a natural function of the aging process. To help prevent or possibly improve this defect, try the far-to-near focus exercise. Hold a pencil about six inches away from your face and focus your eyes on any large object that is 20 to 30 feet away—such as a telephone pole or a flag pole. Then quickly change your focus to the tip of the pencil. Repeatedly switch back and forth between the two objects as quickly as you can— each time focusing as sharply as you are able.

◆ **Eye tracking:** This is an exercise that requires you to keep your head still while following a fast-moving object with the movement of your eyes. Watching a tennis match or watching passing cars is a simple way to do this. While keeping your head still, follow cars moving right to left across your field of vision by tracking them with the movement of your eyes. Then follow the cars moving from left to right across your field of vision. Keep your head as still as possible during this exercise. You might even try balancing a book on your head to assist you in keeping your head still.

◆ **The Bungee Ball:** Here's something all of us can enjoy! This soft rubber ball (about the size of a tennis ball) can be bought at most sporting goods stores. It's attached to

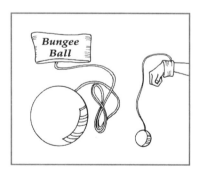

an elasticized cord and has a wristband that prevents it from getting loose. That's why you can have fun with a Bungee Ball even if you're in a wheelchair, or even if you only have use of one hand.

Bungee Balls can be used for exercising the extra-ocular muscles by eye tracking or for far-to-near focus. By swinging it far and near you can do some near-to-closer eye-focusing exercises, and by swinging it side to side you can practice doing eye-tracking exercises—but don't hypnotize yourself!

In terms of improving hand-eye coordination, playing certain sports like tennis, racquetball, or ping-pong is wonderful. But for many of us who can't do this, the Bungee Ball is a good alternative. Because it's attached to a string on your wrist, you can play catch with yourself without having to chase after a loose ball. You can throw it against a wall, throw it from hand to hand, or throw it up in the air and catch it with the same or your opposite hand. Why not give it a try? It's an amusing device that really can improve hand-eye coordination.

LOOKING BACK, LOOKING FORWARD

CHAPTER 14 REVIEW ◆ ◆ ◆

◆ Excellent strength, balance, and endurance exercises can be performed at home.

◆ Since muscles grow when resting (not while exercising), give your muscles some time off by exercising different muscle groups on different days.

◆ At-home exercises for both the upper and lower body can be effectively performed by using only a straight-back chair and a pair of dumbbells (or dumbbell substitutes).

◆ Certain balance exercises can strengthen your gait and help to prevent falls and fractures.

CHAPTER 15 PREVIEW ◆ ◆ ◆

◆ What is "oxygen debt," and how do aerobic exercises help to prevent it?

◆ Why is it important to know my target heart rate (THR) range? How can I use this number as a guide to cardiopulmonary conditioning?

◆ What household activities and recreational sports can provide aerobic endurance training? Is jogging more beneficial than walking?

◆ What must I do to "maintain my gain" in strength and endurance over the long haul?

AEROBIC EXERCISE AND MAINTAINING YOUR GAIN

Our bodies are our gardens/ Our wills are our gardeners.
—William Shakespeare

The word aerobics *came about when the gym
instructors got together and said, "If we're going to
charge $10 an hour, we can't call it jumping up and down."*
—Rita Rudner

OXYGEN DEBT

Do you recall the difference between aerobic and anaerobic exercise that was discussed in chapter 11? Also known as cardio-pulmonary exercise or endurance training, aerobic exercise is designed to improve your cardiopulmonary conditioning by increasing your heart rate for an extended period of time. In large part, this effect is accomplished by carefully paced exercise that avoids creating an *oxygen debt*. You might say it's the *pay as you go* method of working out.

Remember the example I gave of the athlete who sprints 100 yards in 11 seconds? In doing that, he uses up the equivalent of about six liters of oxygen. Although his maximum respiratory quotient (the most oxygen he can inhale) is about four liters a minute—he used six liters in 11 seconds! Because he performed much of the sprint with a reduced oxygen supply to his muscles, he "owes" his body oxygen; he created an *oxygen debt.* That's why you see him panting and gasping for breath after the race—he's paying back the oxygen debt.

AVOIDANCE OF OXYGEN DEBT

Aerobic exercise helps avoid oxygen debt to the greatest extent possible. How? By pacing the exercise so you inhale sufficient oxygen to fuel your muscles and clear the lactate *as you work out.* The exercises that do this best make use of the larger muscles, such as those in our legs and backs. Brisk walking, jogging, and rowing are good examples—as are the exercises done in aerobics classes. Marathon runners and long-distance swimmers are perhaps the best classical examples of advanced aerobic exercisers.

At what point does protracted aerobic exercise eventually enter into an anaerobic phase? When the increased oxygen requirements of the exercising muscles exceed the ability of the cardiopulmonary system to deliver it. That's when oxygen debt develops. How quickly and to what extent this occurs in a given individual varies greatly, depending on that person's muscular and cardiopulmonary conditioning.

What are the three most important factors that determine this efficiency? First, the condition of the lungs determines their ability to transfer inhaled oxygen into the bloodstream. Second, the condition of the heart determines its ability to pump the oxygen-bearing blood to the muscles. And third, the condition of the muscles determines their ability to utilize the oxygen as it's delivered. Think about it. It's easy to see why heart disease, lung disease, and poor muscle conditioning can compromise your ability to do aerobics.

Nonetheless, almost all of us can dramatically improve our conditioning, our endurance, our zest, and our energy by a gradual and progressive approach to aerobics. What about those of us who've been sedentary for so long that our poorly conditioned muscles won't allow us to effectively participate in aerobic exercise? If this is the case, strength training is the first order of business. When our strength is improved, we can go forward by adding endurance training to our program.

FITNESS FOR THE SAKE OF FITNESS VS. FITNESS FOR HEALTH: IS MORE BETTER?

There is no rush. I want you to strive to improve your performance *gradually*. If you rush, you may hurt yourself and end up on the sidelines—and that setback may compromise all the gain you've accomplished. While all of us should try to attain a high level of fitness, there's a level of fitness above which there doesn't appear to be any additional health benefit. This very high level of fitness—which I call *fitness for the sake of fitness*—can be observed in professional athletes such as prizefighters, weightlifters, and marathon runners. Sports injuries are so common in these athletes that attempting to reach that fitness level might, in some cases, be more of a health hazard than a health benefit. Achieving this extraordinary fitness level should be motivated only by love of the sport, as opposed to doing it for added health benefits.

TARGET HEART RATE (THR) RANGE

Many experts believe that aerobic exercise should increase your resting heart rate to your *target heart rate range,* and maintain this level for 20 or 30 minutes, three times a week. Some say this produces a cardiopulmonary health benefit equal to pushing yourself beyond that point—such as a competitive marathon runner would do. *But using the target heart rate range as a guide to effective endurance training is not a great idea for everybody*—and it should always be approached gradually.

Your target heart rate range, or THR range, varies with your age. Here's how to calculate it: The magic starting number is 220. Subtract your age from 220 to determine your maximum heart rate. Then take 75 to 80 percent of that number to determine your THR. As an example, let's say you are 60 years old.

$$\begin{array}{r} 220 \text{ (the magic number)} \\ -\ 60 \text{ (your age)} \\ \hline = 160 \text{ (maximum heart rate)} \end{array}$$

160 heartbeats/minute = maximum heart rate
Never exceed it!

Now take 80 percent of your maximum heart rate.

$$\begin{array}{r} 160 \text{ (maximum heart rate)} \\ \times\ .8 \text{ (80 percent)} \\ \hline = 128 \text{ (THR = target heart rate)} \end{array}$$

That's your THR—128 beats per minute. Again, I advise you not to exceed it, but rather to view it as the upper limit of your target range. The lower limit might be about 10 to 20 beats per minute less. To establish a reasonable range, subtract 10 or 20 from your THR.

Therefore, your THR range = 108 to 128 beats per minute.

If you're 60 years old, your goal during aerobic exercise is to keep your heart beating between 108 and 128 beats per minute for 20 to 30 minutes—and to do it three times a week.

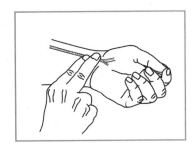

You can count your pulse by applying gentle pressure with the index and middle fingers of one hand to the radial pulse of the opposite wrist. As you practice this, count the number of pulse beats for 20 seconds on your wristwatch and multiply by three. That gives you the number of times your heart is beating each minute. Take your pulse frequently while you are exercising. If you want to go high tech, you can buy a device at some sporting goods stores that will measure your pulse and blood pressure. These gadgets fit on your wrist or on your finger. If you develop shortness of breath or if your heart is beating too fast, slow down or stop for a moment before resuming exercising at a slower pace.

Suppose you're jogging. Do you feel you can carry on a normal conversation with an imaginary person jogging next to you? If not, you're probably entering an anaerobic stage of exercise, and *you're probably developing oxygen debt.* Keep this thought in mind with any of your aerobic endeavors, whether it's bicycling, stair-stepping, jogging, or brisk walking: Judging whether or not you could carry on a conversation is an easy way to identify shortness of breath before it becomes pronounced. If you get chest pain, dizziness, or palpitations during exercise, stop immediately and ask your physician to check it out.

Please understand that it's not your goal to have your heart racing all the time—especially when you're at rest. As your conditioning improves, your resting heart rate will actually get slower. That's because your heart has become more efficient—it can pump more blood with each beat. As an example, it's not at all unusual for a well-conditioned athlete to have a resting pulse rate of 50 to 65 beats per minute.

When you're using the THR range to establish your cardio-pulmonary conditioning, *don't expect to immediately reach and maintain your THR range for 20 minutes.* If you haven't been exercising, it will take time to condition your heart, lungs, and muscles to perform at this level.

IS THE THR ESSENTIAL?

Some of us may be taking a medication that prevents our heart rate from increasing. If that's the case, check with your doctor before starting a program that utilizes THR. Other folks may have an irregular heart rhythm or another longstanding medical condition that could prohibit using this technique. They can still do aerobic exercise to improve their endurance. So while it's not absolutely necessary to use the THR range to improve your endurance, it's an excellent guide to cardiopulmonary conditioning for those of us who can use it and prefer a scientific approach to our workouts.

TREADMILL TESTING, PEAK EXERCISE CAPACITY, AND METABOLIC EQUIVALENTS (METs)

Would you like to get a more precise determination of how fast your own heart *should* beat during exercise? Ask your physician to give you a treadmill test. This could be of considerable importance if you haven't been exercising for a while. The treadmill evaluation can also assess your *peak exercise capacity* measured in units called *metabolic equivalents* or METs. Recent studies suggest that peak exercise capacity, as determined by a treadmill examination and adjusted for age, is probably the best predictor of mortality among men when compared to other established risk factors for cardiovascular disease. If you score in the low range (< 4 METs), your chances of having a serious cardiovascular event are four times higher than if you score in the high range (> 8 METs). Some studies have shown that each 1-MET increase in peak exercise capacity confers a projected 12 percent improvement in survival from a cardiovascular problem. Moreover, your individual MET score can be used as a monitor to gauge your progress. So as your ability to exercise improves, you also improve your MET score, increase your longevity, and enhance your vitality.

HOW TO START AND HOW TO PROGRESS

Regardless of which form of aerobic exercise you choose, start slow, progress gradually, and always remember to stretch and warm up (and gradually cool down) a little both before and after exercising. You might begin by walking or jogging a quarter to a half-mile, and then progress gradually. If you've been a couch potato for a while, you might start by exercising only five minutes a day. That's *okay!* If that is your situation, try to gradually work your way up to 10 minutes for each session, and then try to do two of these sessions a day. Continue to progress until you can do 20 minutes at each session.

When the amount of exercise you're doing seems easy, add a few minutes to your workout every 10 to 20 days until you're doing 30-minute endurance workouts. When this becomes easy, quicken the pace or the difficulty of your exercise a little. For example, if walking is your sport, try walking up a slightly steep hill. You can push yourself a little—but not too much. If you get too short of breath or too fatigued, slow down or stop for a while. And when you finish your workout, don't forget to cool down with a little easy walking and stretching.

THE FREQUENCY OF AEROBIC TRAINING

Some experts think you should be doing some form of exercise for 30 minutes every day. If you're able to do that, I think it's a good idea. But I believe a better plan is *to do endurance training three days a week, strength training at least two days a week, and stretching every day.*

THE BEST EXERCISE

Swimming, rowing, walking, jogging, running, and stair-stepping—as well as some everyday activities—qualify as good endurance training exercises. You can get an endurance workout mowing the lawn, raking leaves, or mopping the floor. Each activity has some advantages and some drawbacks, and each of you will find or develop your own preferences. Let's talk a little about some of them.

Swimming and aquabatics

Swimming can be a great aerobic exercise, and it also improves your strength. For many, it's also very enjoyable and refreshing, and because it's a low-impact exercise, it's not likely to injure your joints. Equally important, because of the buoyancy provided by the water, excessive body weight doesn't compromise one's ability to work out. This can be of particular value to people who are obese. The buoyancy factor also facilitates stretching and doing some lower-body resistance training. (Exercising in the pool is often termed *aquabatics* or *aquaerobics*.)

Most of us, however, are not excellent swimmers. This lack of expertise can compromise our chances of getting a good cardio-pulmonary workout by swimming. Our strokes and our kicks are less than perfect, and our breathing technique is usually poor. As a result, many of us find ourselves gasping for breath before we've had a really good workout. If you're a very good swimmer, swimming can be a wonderful way to combine aerobics with strength training and stretching. But even in this case, one of its advantages is also a disadvantage: Swimming is a low-impact exercise. While this decreases the chances of joint injury, it does less than some other exercises to prevent osteoporosis or increase bone mineral density. To get this benefit, we need greater stress on our bones or a moderate amount of impact in our exercise program.

Stair-stepping

For most of us, stair-stepping is a better aerobics choice than swimming. Why? You don't have to be a good swimmer to do this. You can climb up and down an ordinary flight of stairs, or you can use a stair-stepping machine. There are many variations in stair-stepping machines, including some that work your arms at the same time you're working your legs. You can get an excellent aerobic workout with this exercise in addition to some strength-training benefit to both your upper and lower body. But stair-stepping is much more of an aerobic workout than a strength-training activity. Here again, it's a low-impact exercise that protects your joints—but it has a lesser effect on improving bone density.

Walking and biking

Now let's talk a little about walking and bike riding. Most of us can safely enjoy walking, and some of us can go biking as well. You can pick a safe and pleasant place to walk or bike and enjoy the sights while getting a nice workout, or you can use a treadmill or stationary bike in front of a TV screen. A brisk walk for 45 to 60 minutes will burn about 100 calories per mile. So if you walk three or three and a half miles, you can burn 300 or more calories and get a good aerobic workout. But the walk has to be brisk—not a window-shopping type of stroll. This is important to keep in mind if you do your walking at shopping malls.

If you walk three and a half miles in an hour, you're covering a mile every 17 to 18 minutes—a nice clip. Many of us can't do that to start. We may be able to walk only a quarter of a mile—about once around the block or once around the outside perimeter of a football field. As always, start slow and gradually increase your distance before increasing your speed.

Many treadmills have an adjustable incline. That means you can increase the difficulty of the exercise as well as the speed. Some of the more sophisticated treadmill machines and stationary bikes also have pulse meters and calorie counters. These can be of great assistance to those of us who want to use the THR range to monitor pulse rate and caloric expenditure while we're working out.

Bear in mind that these are low-impact exercises such as swimming and stair-stepping, and while walking and biking are excellent methods of cardiopulmonary conditioning, they, too, do less to enhance bone density than jogging, running, or resistance training. Don't get me wrong—they're all excellent endurance training activities. They may even have a positive influence on bone mineral density. However, if they are the *only* exercises you do, I suggest you consider jogging in place for a minute or two after your workout. The impact provided by this simple add-on movement might help to strengthen your bones.

Jogging and jog-breaking

Jogging and running are very popular high-impact exercises. Both are excellent cardiopulmonary exercises that can have a significantly positive effect on bone mineral density. Their downside is the possibility of joint injury from the constant jarring that attends these activities (ankles, knees, hips, and low back). So start these activities slowly and progress slowly—particularly if you've been sedentary. If you fall into this category, one way to get started is to begin with brisk walking. After you're comfortable doing this, try a "jog-break"—interrupt your walk every five minutes with 10 or 20 seconds of jogging. After you've done this for a week or two, try jogging for 30 to 60 seconds every five minutes. As your conditioning improves, you can progressively increase the amount of jogging and decrease the amount of walking until, voila!—you're jogging! And if you want to run, simply go faster. These are all wonderful and highly addicting endeavors. But please remember that *gradual* is the operative word—*progress gradually.*

Aerobics classes

Most of the better aerobics programs are divided into beginner, intermediate, and advanced classes. These classes are often a lot of fun and are commonly characterized by a great deal of energy and enthusiasm. They encourage a sense of social intercourse and individual as well as group achievement. Yet despite this benefit, many aerobics classes fail to address the specific needs of the individual participants. Each of us—especially in the beginner class—has a different level of fitness. Those of us at a lower level are sometimes unwittingly seduced into trying to keep up with the group (our competitive nature in action). On one hand, this can be motivating. On the other hand, however, some people might work out a little harder than they should and do some things they shouldn't—

resulting in injury. I've seen this happen a number of times. If aerobics classes are your thing, keep these issues in mind. Aerobics classes can be wonderful, but be sure your instructor is knowledgeable and attentive to your individual state of fitness. If he or she is not, find a different instructor.

INTERRELATION OF ENDURANCE AND STRENGTH TRAINING

Endurance training and strength training are not mutually exclusive—in fact, just the opposite; they're as interrelated as the horse and carriage! If you have a marked decrease in muscle strength, you cannot perform endurance training exercises effectively. As previously mentioned, if this is your situation, strength training is the first order of business for you. Clearly, when you've improved your strength, your endurance will also be improved. At this point, if you use some of the endurance-training techniques already discussed to further improve your staying power, your strength-training program will also benefit. You'll be able to use more resistance and do more for a longer period of time. Or you can combine a strength-training workout with an aerobics workout by circuit training.

COMBINING STRENGTH TRAINING AND AEROBICS BY CIRCUIT TRAINING

If you've been strength training and you're beginning to shape up, you can modify your strength-training sessions to include a good cardiopulmonary workout. This can be achieved by *circuit training*—going from one resistance exercise to the next after just one set. Do this by decreasing the resistance, increasing the number of reps, and decreasing the rest periods between your circuit of exercises. Here's how:

- ◆ Reduce the weight/resistance that you use in your usual workout by 50 percent or more for each resistance exercise.

- ◆ Do just one set of each resistance exercise—but increase the number of reps in each exercise, with the lighter weight, from your usual 8 or 12 reps to 15 or even 25 reps.

- ◆ As you go from one resistance exercise to the next, decrease the rest periods between resistance exercises to 30 seconds or even down to 10 seconds.

- ◆ Continue to repeat the circuit until you've worked out for 30 minutes.

Remember that spending more time exercising your larger muscles (such as the leg and back muscles) is likely to give you a better cardiopulmonary workout than working smaller muscles (such as your biceps or triceps). So, to combine strength with endurance conditioning, work a little more on the leg press, leg extension, leg curl, and back machines.

INTERRUPTIONS

Suppose you have to interrupt your workout schedule for a couple of weeks. Be sure to resume your exercise program slowly. *Don't expect to pick up where you left off right away.* For the first week that you're back at it, start with half the resistance you've been using for strength training, and do half the amount of endurance training you usually do. Then increase it to 75 percent for the second week. From there on, gradually increase your workouts to your prior level.

You *will* get there. Don't panic. There's no rush. If for some reason, you lay off for two or three months, you can lose the gain you've achieved and may have to start again from scratch. This kind of layoff may be unavoidable because of illness, but *don't let this cause you to abandon exercise—stay with it.* If, for whatever reason, a long lapse does occur, think of how good you felt when you were fit, and *start again.* Don't be disheartened.

OVERWORK

Occasionally our muscles seem to need more rest or recuperative time. This is particularly true among some older adults—but it can happen to anyone at any age. Often, but not always, this follows an unusually strenuous workout. In these cases, 48 hours may not be enough time for our muscles to repair and ready themselves for the next effort. When we try to work them out again, we find that we perform less well than we did on our prior workout. When this happens, it's easy to get depressed and come to believe that we're regressing or failing to progress. *Don't get down in the mouth about this.* Why? Because this, too, is normal. Give yourself a longer rest. Take 72 hours off and start again. If you still find yourself on a continuing downward slope—or if you experience dizziness, chest pain, or palpitations when you exercise—see your doctor for a checkup.

THE CHALLENGE: MAINTAINING THE GAIN IN STRENGTH AND ENDURANCE

If you've been sedentary, it's common to see significant improvement in your ability to work out and your "feeling of fitness" in just one month. After that, improvement is likely to be slower and peak after 8 to 12 weeks. Most of us will continue to improve—but our progress will probably be more gradual than the dramatic difference we achieved in the first 12 weeks. You might also note that some workouts and some weeks are better than others—or that your performance today is less than it was a week ago. If so, don't be discouraged. These variations can be normal and don't necessarily mean that you're regressing. There can be many reasons for an occasional slow-down—such as a long layoff from working out because of illness, travel, etc. It may be that you've been working out too hard or too much, and you haven't allowed sufficient time for your muscles to recuperate.

While your capacity to continually improve is in part defined by your age, in part by your dedication, and in part by your genetic makeup, your goal is to do what it takes to maintain the better level of fitness you've achieved. To maintain strength, most people establish a routine of a designated number of reps and sets with a designated resistance (discussed in previous chapters). For cardiopulmonary maintenance, they perform endurance exercises a certain number of times each week at a specific level of intensity over a designated period of time. But many people find that by sticking with an exercise maintenance program that is consistently non-progressive, they actually enter a regressive stage. In other words, your same old maintenance program becomes increasingly more difficult to perform, and sometimes results in regression!

The best way to avoid this problem and to *maintain your gains* is to challenge yourself on a regularly scheduled basis. For example, I've found it useful to challenge my routine once every 10 to 14 days by slightly increasing the weight or resistance I use for one set of each of the movements in my strength-training exercises. Alternatively, once every two weeks or so, you might try increasing the number of reps in a set or two. I also try to slightly increase the difficulty or length of my usual endurance exercise once every ten days to two weeks. I believe that creating these small, occasional challenges can help maintain the integrity of an ongoing maintenance program.

LOOKING BACK, LOOKING FORWARD

CHAPTER 15 REVIEW • • •

◆ Aerobics provides excellent endurance training by conditioning the heart, lungs, and muscles.

◆ Low-impact forms of aerobic exercises include swimming, walking, stair-stepping, and biking. High-impact forms include jogging and jog-breaking.

◆ Calculating your target heart rate (THR) range can provide an excellent guide to cardiopulmonary conditioning.

◆ Varying your exercise routines can help you maintain your gains in endurance and strength.

CHAPTER 16 PREVIEW • • •

◆ Is it possible to maintain a satisfying sex life in spite of advancing age? What role is played by decreasing hormones?

◆ Can improving your physical fitness also improve your sex life? How can better communication overcome fear of failure?

◆ What are some personal hygiene challenges we may face as we age?

◆ How does personal hygiene relate to dignity, self-esteem, and "aging gracefully"?

SEXUAL ACTIVITY AND PERSONAL HYGIENE IN THE OLDER ADULT

*Love is the answer—but while you're waiting for
the answer, sex raises some pretty good questions.*

—Woody Allen

I think making love is the best form of exercise.

—Cary Grant

SEX AND THE OLDER ADULT

Would it surprise you to know that, for many, sex actually becomes even more pleasurable with age? Maybe it's because we have fewer pressures such as work deadlines, keeping appointments, the fear of pregnancy, and the like. Even in nursing homes, romantic relationships develop that may culminate in sexual activity. Many compassionate attendants learn to look the other way, and some establishments even provide a comfortable surrounding for these events. Others prohibit them, and even chastise the residents for these consensual interludes. This isn't to say that our sexual function remains unchanged as we get older; it doesn't. But a better understanding of these changes—as well as how you might deal with them—can help prevent disappointment or despair.

FREQUENCY

Most of you don't need to be told that there really is sex after 40. In fact, there's even sex after 80! About 60 percent of men and women between the ages of 40 and 60 engage in some form of sexual activity about once a week. More than 25 percent of people 75 and older also have sex almost once a week. With advancing age and declining health, the frequency and type of sexual activity varies from once a week to three or four times a year to none at all.

Under such circumstances, loving relationships and cuddling—while always important—become even *more* important. What factors discourage sexual activity? Depression, chronic pain, general unfitness, a lack of communication, hormonal changes, medications, erectile dysfunction, and a host of other issues all combine to diminish libido and decrease sexual activity.

LIBIDO

The term "libido" refers to sexual desire—the appetite for sex. To some extent, libido varies with gender. One study, for example, has shown that men think about sex on an average of once an hour, and women think about it perhaps two or three times a day. We have to be careful about how we interpret this data. It only suggests that it's more frequently on the minds of men—not necessarily that women enjoy sex less.

INTRINSIC HORMONAL CHANGES

What are the things that affect libido, and what can we do about them? Let's discuss these issues from two standpoints: *intrinsic factors* and *extrinsic factors*. By intrinsic factors, I am referring to hormonal changes. There can be no doubt that sex hormones decrease as we age. Postmenopausal women produce significantly less estrogen than their younger counterparts, and older men produce significantly less testosterone. In women, this can result in emotional changes associated with a waning libido, loss of energy, and a decrease in vaginal lubrication. In men, the decrease in testosterone may also be associated with a decrease in libido, lack of fitness, and erectile dysfunction.

Vaginal lubricants and estrogen therapy (in selected cases) can be very effective for some women. Less often, testosterone therapy can be partially effective in some men. I say *partially effective* because in most instances the major impediments to sexual activity are due to a potpourri of extrinsic factors and only partially due to the intrinsic hormonal deficiencies.

EXTRINSIC FACTORS:
Depression and medications
Chronic depression, medications, and the fear of failure loom high on the list of causes for sexual difficulties. It's a fact that many medications used to treat depression may adversely affect libido. Some other medications—used to treat everything from ulcers to high blood pressure—can also diminish the sexual appetite, and some can even cause erectile dysfunction. The list of these agents is too long to get into here.

So, if you're taking medicine and having trouble with your sexual appetite or trouble getting or maintaining an erection, check with your doctor about a possible cause-and-effect relationship.

On another note: You might recall from reading Shakespeare that alcohol can increase your libido but also decrease your sexual performance. So, if it's love you choose, don't over-booze.

Fear of failure

All of you guys and gals who are reading this know what I mean when I talk about the "fear of failure." Every man will, at one time or another, experience impotence and be unable to get an erection. Occasional incidents are not abnormal and may result from fatigue, worry, depression, or anxiety. These intermittent episodes are not necessarily a sign of weakening sexual ability; *from time to time, they occur in almost everybody.* However, a disappointing episode can sometimes be so traumatic it creates a level of anxiety that perpetuates even more fear of failure. The important thing is to understand it for what it is. *It's temporary; it's not abnormal; it's not a disease.* The best remedy is to stop worrying and get on with your fun.

A similar phenomenon can occur with the ladies. You may be used to having orgasms on a regular basis, and then—one, two, or more times in a row this fails to happen. Perhaps you become convinced that it's over—you'll never have another orgasm. That thought may be so disappointing that you become depressed. Don't fall into this trap! This can happen to any woman from time to time. It also can be the result of anxiety, worry, or even because you're not feeling well as a result of an illness. At other times, it's caused by a lack of communication between you and your lover, or perhaps boredom with the love-making technique. If you're not satisfied, talk about it and try to work it out. Try different approaches or different positions. Discuss your fantasies with your partner. Under these circumstances, there's no substitute for candor. But to avoid hurt feelings, the candor should be delivered with care. If this doesn't work, consider consulting a specialist in the field.

Chronic disease and chest pain

All of us know that making love requires a significant amount of exertion—exertion that can cause some shortness of breath, if you do it right. Chronic lung disease that compromises breathing can aggravate this situation to the extent that sexual activity becomes undesirable or even impossible. The same can be said for congestive heart failure and for unstable angina. Chest pain caused by the exertion of lovemaking can be frightening and make the very thought of sex undesirable and even dangerous. If you are so afflicted, it's important that you check with your doctor. He or she may be able to treat these problems so that sex can once again be an enjoyable and safe part of your life.

Unfitness

Lack of fitness is a different issue. Some people are simply so out of shape or so obese that they don't have the physical stamina for sex—so they convince themselves that they're no longer interested. But getting fit will not only make us look sexier, it will make us *be* sexier! That means exercise, eating right, and quitting smoking. You'll have more stamina, more desire, more zest for life, and more fun—and your partner will, too. In this regard, the resistance training, the endurance training, and the stretching exercises we've discussed are very important. As an example: If you're more flexible you will have greater ease of motion. In other words, if you improve your flexibility you may increase your sex-ability. When you do start enjoying sex again, don't delude yourself by imagining that sexual activity is a substitute for regular exercise—because it isn't. Even vigorous sexual activity only burns about two calories a minute.

PAINFUL SEX

Painful sex, in both males and females, must be divided into two categories. One is pain in the genital area during intercourse, and the other is pain outside the genital area. It's important to distinguish between the two.

Genital pain

Both men and women can experience pain in the genital areas during sexual intercourse. This is somewhat more common among women and is sometimes the result of a urinary tract infection or inadequate vaginal lubrication. Some men just don't allow their partners enough time to be sufficiently aroused, or perhaps they don't do enough gentle petting before attempting penile insertion. Listen up, guys! *Haste can hurt your partner.* So take your time and be gentle.

Some gentle sexual petting can do a lot to increase vaginal lubrication and elasticity. This can set the stage for a much more enjoyable experience for the both of you. Even though natural vaginal lubrication can decrease with advancing age, it is easily remedied with the use of vaginal lubricants applied before sex. You can find such products in any drug store, or ask your doctor for a recommendation. (But again, guys, don't use such lubricants as a substitute for the loving arousal of your partner.)

Men can also experience discomfort in the genital area when having sex. Usually, this is the result of an irritation or an infection in this region. An inflammation of the urinary bladder or the urethra (the tube that leads outward from the bladder through the shaft of the penis) can cause discomfort during sex or even when passing urine.

Pain on ejaculation can be experienced as a result of an inflammation of the prostate gland or the seminal vesicles—the pouches that hold and empty semen during ejaculation. Often, the cause of these conditions can be quickly diagnosed and cured, so make a trip to your doctor.

Pain outside the genital area

People with arthritis, low back pain, and chronic abdominal discomfort are often limited in many of their activities, including sex. For those with chronic arthritis or low back discomfort, taking their anti-inflammatory medication prior to making love will often permit a more enjoyable experience. Also, abdominal discomfort or low back discomfort during sex can sometimes be avoided. How? By trying positions other than the missionary position—we'll talk more about this shortly.

And while the subjects of hormone replacement therapy, erection, and erectile dysfunction, as well as disorders of the prostate gland, are extremely important, they are more thoroughly discussed in chapter 17.

CONNECTILE DYSFUNCTION

Now, I'd like to address what I've come to call "connectile dysfunction"—some of the issues that make us sexually attracted to each other or, on the other hand, turn us off.

ROMANCE

Let's spend a little time discussing the idea of romance. I'm not talking about reciting poetry (although sometimes that could be a very good idea, too). Many of you know the wisdom of remembering birthdays and anniversaries with a little gift of flowers or cologne. This is all very important. It can even be a good idea, once in awhile, to buy some cute or sexy lingerie. Whether the man sometimes buys it for his partner or the lady buys it herself, believe me, it can add a little spice to your life.

Demeanor and communication

What contributed to the fun of your youth? Examine the features of your courtships that made them successful. These are things that some of us forget or take for granted as we get a little older. Or perhaps we mistakenly believe they aren't as important as they once were. Some examples: your approach to your partner, your communication techniques, your manners, and your appearance—even your state of cleanliness and the smell of your skin. All these factors can go a long way toward enhancing the pleasure of your relationship.

Many men assume that when they're ready, their partner is also ready. But the sword of Alexander the Great—your proud erection—is not the equivalent of a bugle sounding the charge of the Light Brigade. Be a tad patient. Don't scare your partner. Indulge in kissing and petting before thrusting yourself upon her like the alpha gorilla we men sometimes envision ourselves to be. Develop a form of communication, either verbal or by touch, that both of you recognize and can respond to. Your partner may not be feeling well or for some other reason be unable to enjoy sex at that time. *Both of you must learn to accept that without getting angry.*

If poor timing is an ongoing event, have a candid discussion about the issue. But make sure that it's not an argument or a blaming session. It should be a gentle and constructive effort on the part of both partners. Most problems have solutions—and in this case, both partners must participate in developing them.

Personal hygiene

Apart from its influence on sexuality, personal hygiene is important from a health standpoint. While most of us appreciate the importance of cleanliness, some of us older folk become lax and place less emphasis on it than we should. Think about it: This is often because we don't care about ourselves as much as we once did. Perhaps we've lost our sense of importance and our self-esteem. In other instances, we're just downright lazy. Frankly, some of us don't bathe as frequently as we should.

Not only does dirt represent a real health hazard, but esthetically, nothing can turn off your partner more quickly than poor hygiene. So bathe or shower at least once every day and put on clean socks and clean underwear every day as well. And try the daily application of a good moisturizing body lotion to help keep your skin from drying out and flaking.

We're not very good at smelling ourselves, so don't bother sniffing your armpit to determine whether or not you need to bathe or shower. Trust me—if you don't clean yourself, you're gonna stink. You may not know it, but everybody else will. Our olfactory senses, the nerve endings in the nose that detect odors, quickly become accustomed to our own odor. As an example, when you put on some cologne or perfume, in a very short while you don't notice it, do you? But others can smell it. This is because your sense of smell accommodates quickly—within minutes.

Also, as we age, our sense of smell isn't as sharp as it was when we were younger. That's no doubt why some of you charming ladies put on entirely too much perfume. Not infrequently, older women and some men splash on so much of the stuff that they literally reek! Be aware, my friends, that our sense of smell deteriorates with age—so don't go too heavy on the cologne or perfume.

Some older adults take too few baths or showers because they fear slipping or falling. In many cases, this is a reasonable concern. But that can usually be dealt with by making the bath or shower safer—with rails, seats, and slip-retardant mats or tiles. Another alternative, one that many couples find pleasantly effective, is to use the buddy system for bathing or showering.

What could be more bonding than helping each other wash while you also protect each other from falling?

Toilet hygiene and oral hygiene

In addition to bathing, the special issue of toilet hygiene must be addressed. There are two ends to be tended to: brushing your teeth and cleaning yourself after a bowel movement.

Sour breath is a big industry. Hundreds and hundreds of breath mints and other remedies for bad breath are for sale in stores and over hotlines. Why? Superb marketing has rather successfully produced mass paranoia. These marketing techniques are geared to convince the public that everybody needs these things because everybody has bad breath. To some extent, that's true. At one time or another everybody does have foul-smelling breath. And you can't really smell your own breath no matter how hard you try, or whatever hand-cupping techniques you might employ. Remember—you can't smell yourself.

No doubt these breath mints and chewing gums can be refreshing from time to time. So if you enjoy them, have at it. But that doesn't mean you should become paranoid and suck or eat a handful of breath mints every few hours. It's much more important to have a clean mouth, healthy teeth, and healthy gums. This is best accomplished by flossing and brushing your teeth after each meal and seeing your dentist on a regular basis—the most effective assurance of clean breath and a healthy mouth. I know it's not always convenient, but certainly most of us can brush our teeth at least twice a day. Breath mints are okay—but they're not a substitute for good oral hygiene.

Dentures can cause a bad breath problem. Usually this can be well-controlled with proper cleaning of the dentures and the use of any one of a number of pleasant-tasting mouthwashes on the market.

Perianal cleansing

On an even more delicate subject—some of us, as we age, aren't as careful as we should be about cleaning ourselves after a bowel movement. What could be more of a turnoff than residual fecal material still clinging to your body? It's important to clean yourself carefully and thoroughly. This doesn't mean that you should scrub yourself raw—that's the wrong thing to do. The skin around the perianal area is tender and should be treated tenderly. Vigorous scrubbing can irritate the skin and set it up for an infection. A good technique is to gently swab the area with moistened toilet paper until it is clean, and then blot it with dry toilet paper. I appreciate that some folks may have difficulty reaching back there because of physical limitations that may have been acquired over the years. In these cases, cleansing might be more efficient if you use some of those pre-moistened, flushable anal wipes. You can buy them at almost any drug store.

Gaseousness

Another delicate subject is intestinal gas. Everyone has intestinal gas, and all of us have excessive intestinal gas from time to time. In some people, it's more of a problem than it is to others. Occasionally, excess gaseousness causes us to burp or "butt burp"—a very understandable situation. Most partners use humor and an understanding of the other partner's distress to accommodate each other's need to seek relief.

Some people, however, unnecessarily allow themselves to expel gas at inappropriate times. To hear some of my patients tell it, their bed has become a farting field. Their spouses actually wait to get into bed before erupting. Sometimes these eruptions are silent and full of odiferous surprises; at other times, they're a symphony of broken trumpets. For some reason, the offenders come to believe that their partners are used to it—so it doesn't matter. In a few cases that may be true, but in most others, it has a very negative conscious or even unconscious effect on the romance of your bed—where you sleep, dream, and make love.

If you do this, do what you can to break the habit. Look back through earlier chapters for some of the causes and remedies for excessive gaseousness. If they don't work for you, consult your doctor. He or she might be able to help.

Appearance

We don't need to hide our age—but we sure don't have to *advertise* it, either! Wearing neckties, shirts, dresses, or pants with food spots and possibly even urine stains suggests that you don't care about personal hygiene. If you're dirty on the outside, it seems reasonable to assume that you're probably dirty down under—that you have dirty socks and underwear on and that your body is dirty. That's *not* aging gracefully!

Presenting a slovenly appearance diminishes your dignity and projects a lack of self-esteem. There's no reason why men can't shave or keep a beard neatly groomed or maintain a head of nicely trimmed and combed hair.

The same cautions apply to women. Some ladies apply makeup like war masks—perhaps because they don't see as well as they used to. Sometimes it's so thick that it drips onto the collar of their clothing. At other times, it really *is* a mask because it stops at the chin instead of being blended lower. My advice is to get a better magnifying mirror, apply a little less makeup, and blend it in carefully. And never ever use cosmetics as a substitute for cleanliness.

You are an important person. You deserve to look like you care about yourself. If we don't care about ourselves, others won't care either. This is all part of aging gracefully.

THE SEX ACT

To complete our discussion of this subject, let's say a few words about the sex act itself, which can sometimes become a little more challenging in older adults. Physical and mental limitations—such as arthritis, heart disease, lung disease, erectile dysfunction, depression, and so on—can obviously have an impact on the physical act. But any one, or even a combination of such limitations, does *not* have to mean an end to your physical sex life. You just need to be a little more creative—and a lifetime of experience has made us ready to meet this challenge!

Foreplay

Let's be realistic; those youthful encounters in the backseat of a car no longer generate the excitement they did when they were *forbidden*. And while a spontaneous "roll in the hay" is always fun, we now have the time and the luxury of being able to

312

participate in extended foreplay—perhaps dinner, a nightcap in front of the fireplace, cuddling and caressing, and maybe even some of that backseat heavy petting. Foreplay is almost always an important beginning to a mutually satisfying encounter.

And what if this encounter—for whatever reason—doesn't result in intercourse? Hopefully, you've had a great time and achieved emotional satisfaction that will be remembered until your next encounter.

The best foreplay of all is the way you treat each other in your daily lives! I'm talking about things like caring for each other, talking with each other, laughing together, always greeting each other with a smile, a hug, and a kiss, and *never taking each other for granted*. The love, care, and respect you put into your relationship on a daily basis is an aphrodisiac that will enhance your life for years to come.

Positions for sex

A variety of sexual positions can accommodate some of the physical limitations we've discussed. (But even if you are free of physical limitations, remember that "variety is the spice of life!")

The so-called *missionary position* is one that everybody understands. It's best described as the woman on the bottom and the man on top, with the female partner's legs spread and the legs of the male partner between those of the female.

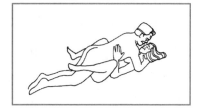

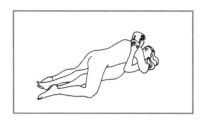

A simple variation of this position is as follows: After insertion of the penis into the vagina, the male puts his legs outside those of the female as the female partner slowly brings her legs inside the legs of her male partner. This position might prove more comfortable for some partners—especially those with hip problems—or it may provide an enjoyable variation for others.

A reversal of the missionary position with the female partner on top can be particularly useful for couples when the male partner has low back problems or the female partner has a tender abdomen.

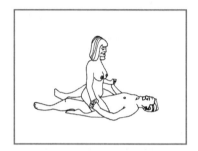

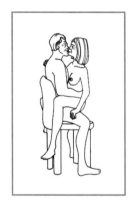

Another variation for men with low back discomfort is the *sitting on a chair position*. In this situation, the male partner sits on a chair and the female partner straddles the thighs of the male partner.

Many people (somewhat more commonly females) suffer from chronic abdominal discomfort. Sometimes this is the result of pelvic surgery and the development of adhesions—as might occur following a hysterectomy or appendectomy. Sometimes it's due to chronic constipation or excessive gaseousness. Men have to take their partners' discomfort into consideration. Imagine the terror of seeing some big guy about to jump on *your* sore belly!

Still another position, one that might ameliorate or decrease a woman's abdominal discomfort during intercourse, is the so-called *stallion on the mare position*. In this position the female partner is

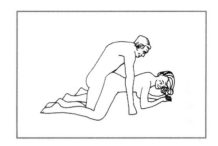

on her hands and knees (or on her elbows and knees) and the male partner assumes a position behind her. She can get some additional support by stacking two or three pillows beneath her

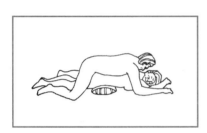

lower abdomen and pelvis. The male partner is then able to insert his penis into the vagina from the rear, which avoids putting the pressure of his weight on the abdomen of his female partner.

Now there are many other positions that you might like to try. If you're interested in more ideas, you can find a good sex manual in almost any bookstore or at your local library.

Oral sexual relationships

I think it's important to say a few words about oral-genital relationships. Some may view this negatively—but you would be surprised at how many older adults really enjoy these pleasures. The important factors here are twofold: *cleanliness* and *consensuality.* Good personal hygiene and cleanliness can make this activity pleasurable—and poor personal hygiene can make it a really bad experience, to say the least. Most importantly, the activity must be consensual. Forcing or requiring your partner to indulge in an activity that he or she considers undesirable can be a real turnoff.

Sexually transmitted diseases (STDs)

These diseases are less common in older adults because relationships are more likely to be monogamous. But make no mistake about it: Older adults with multiple sexual partners are definitely at risk. *Everyone* should be certain to practice safe sex, use condoms, and wash carefully.

LOOKING BACK, LOOKING FORWARD

CHAPTER 16 REVIEW ◆ ◆ ◆

◆ By adapting to changing circumstances, older adults can and do continue to have enjoyable sexual relationships.

◆ Chronic depression, some medications, fear of failure, and physical limitations are causes of sexual difficulties that should be discussed with your doctor.

◆ Self-care in the form of cleanliness and care for appearance helps maintain dignity and self-esteem—critical factors in "aging gracefully."

◆ To promote mutually satisfying sexual relationships, the influence of hygiene, appearance, romance, demeanor, and communication cannot be overstated.

CHAPTER 17 PREVIEW ◆ ◆ ◆

◆ What kind of medications best control the symptoms of prostate gland enlargement?

◆ Does prostate surgery always result in sexual impotency?

◆ How is erectile dysfunction (ED) best treated?

◆ What are the advantages and disadvantages of hormone replacement therapy (HRT)?

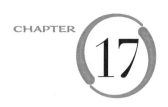

THE PROSTATE GLAND, ERECTILE DYSFUNCTION, AND HORMONE REPLACEMENT

It is much more important to know what sort of patient has a disease than to know what sort of a disease a patient has.
—William Osler

Do what you can, with what you have, where you are.
—Theodore Roosevelt

THE PROSTATE GLAND

The prostate gland is normally about the size of a chestnut, but it can enlarge to the size of a big orange. Composed of glandular material and strands of muscle, the prostate gland surrounds the first inch or so of the urethra at its junction with the bladder. Some of the muscle fibers in the prostate gland blend with the muscle fibers of the bladder at this junction. While the prostate doesn't produce any hormones, its glandular elements secrete a

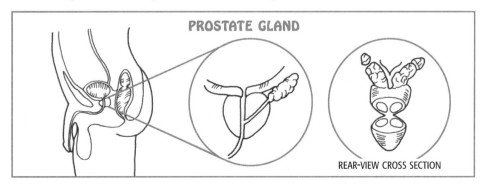

PROSTATE GLAND

REAR-VIEW CROSS SECTION

fluid that, together with the fluid of the seminal vesicles, is added to the sperm during ejaculation. Most of the back side of the gland, being situated in front of the rectum, can easily be felt during a rectal examination.

BENIGN PROSTATIC HYPERPLASIA (BPH)

A condition called *benign prostatic hyperplasia* or BPH is the most common cause of prostate gland enlargement. Prostate *cancer* is an entirely different condition that will be addressed in the next chapter. In BPH, the term *hyperplasia* is used to indicate an increase in the number of cells in the prostate gland. This condition can cause anything from a mild to a massive enlargement of the gland.

What happens when the prostate becomes enlarged? It, along with spasticity of the prostatic musculature, encroaches on the urethra and impedes the flow of urine. This can produce a myriad of unpleasant symptoms. The obstruction to urinary flow results in incomplete evacuation of the bladder, which in turn causes urinary frequency throughout the day and may even disturb your sleep with the need to void several times during the night. You might also experience any or all of the following symptoms: difficulty in starting urination, diminished size and force of your urinary stream, post-urinary dribbling, or even an overflow dribbling. Excruciating urinary urgency and bladder distension may become a problem—especially if *acute urinary retention* occurs. On rare occasions, this can happen without warning, but it is usually precipitated by repeatedly denying the urge to void or taking some seemingly innocuous medications that can aggravate urinary retention. Some "likely suspects" among such medications are bowel relaxants (anticholinergics), decongestants, and antihistamines.

When total obstruction to urinary flow occurs (as in acute urinary retention), emergency measures in the form of catheterization or even surgery may be necessary. To make matters worse, the chronic retention of urine can predispose you to recurrent urinary tract infections and damage your urinary bladder. Over time, the progressive stretching of the bladder wall can weaken the wall and may even result in the formation of pockets or out-pouchings called *bladder diverticuli.*

THE CAUSE OF BPH

The reasons BPH occurs more often with advancing age are not entirely clear. Microscopic studies on prostate gland tissue have shown that hyperplasia increases in frequency from eight percent in men from 31 to 40 years old, to 50 percent in men from 51 to 60 years old, to more than 80 percent in men older than 80. Here's the puzzle: We know that testosterone increases the growth of the prostate, and we know that testosterone production decreases with advancing age. Therefore, we would expect advancing age to *decrease* the size of the prostate gland rather than increase it.

Some investigators theorize that the threshold of prostatic tissue for the action of testosterone is lowered as age advances to an extent that more than compensates for the diminished production of the male hormone. Others postulate that the conversion of testosterone to dihydrotestosterone (DHT), which is the active form of the hormone responsible for prostatic growth, is increased. Still others speculate that prostatic hyperplasia results from an imbalance between estrogen and testosterone that occurs with aging. Simply stated, *it happens, and we just don't know why*. Hopefully, ongoing research will give us some answers in the near future.

TREATMENT AND PRECAUTIONARY MEASURES

The treatment your doctor recommends will, in large part, be determined by the severity of your symptoms, the size of your gland, your age, and the presence or absence of other complicating diseases—so-called *comorbid conditions*. With less than severe symptoms and with mild to moderate enlargement of the gland, you will probably do very well with medical therapy.

If you experience a sudden increase in urgency or frequency, or if you develop burning on urination or blood in your urine, your condition is most likely complicated by a urinary tract infection (UTI). See your doctor if this occurs. He or she may recommend a urine culture and prescribe antibiotics.

Let me suggest some commonsense precautionary measures that can reduce the distress associated with BPH. Urinary frequency can be reduced by avoiding those things that promote excessive urination, such as alcohol or beverages containing caffeine (tea, coffee, etc.). Surprisingly, many soft drinks contain large amounts of caffeine, so read labels carefully. You might also save yourself a few wakeup calls if you avoid drinking beverages near bedtime.

Many of my patients have described an even worse scenario such as being seized by a painful and almost undeniable need to urinate when you're stuck in a traffic jam. Try to anticipate this or similar problems by making it a habit to urinate before leaving your home or place of business. And don't forget that certain medications (anticholinergics, decongestants, antihistamines, etc.) can aggravate these symptoms or even precipitate acute urinary retention in patients with BPH. I've known patients who were catapulted to the emergency room after taking a seemingly harmless cold remedy that contained a decongestant or antihistamine. However, some of the newer antihistamine drugs are much less likely to cause such a reaction. So if you have BPH and need to take antihistamines, please check with your doctor. Before leaving this subject, there's another bit of advice I'd like to give all of you fastidious gentlemen. It goes like this:

Before you zip,   *If you close your fly*
 please be hip.   *before you're dry,*
Shake your tip   *You'll be a sticky guy*
 to shed that drip.   *with an icky thigh.*

Medications that can help

When the prostate gland isn't too large, disturbing symptoms and progressive damage to the urinary bladder can often be controlled with the use of medications called *alpha-adrenergic blockers*—such as Hytrin, Cardura, Flomax, and others. These medications can relax the musculature of the prostate and allow for an easier egress of urine out of the bladder. In other words, they help open the gate that's guarded by the prostate's spastic musculature around the first inch or two of the urethra.

Some other medications have been effective in decreasing the symptoms of BPH by arresting the growth or even reducing the size of the prostate. They work by blocking the conversion of testosterone to dihydrotestosterone (Proscar and Avodart). Some studies have suggested they adversely affect sexual function—libido, potency, and the volume of the ejaculate. Other studies show that these effects are no more frequent than they are with placebos. On the downside, these medications can artificially lower blood PSA determinations, which makes a very important screening test for prostate cancer less useful. Moreover, unlike the alpha-blockers, Proscar and Avodart take time to work. You have to be patient.

Some European studies have suggested that saw palmetto, an herb extracted from the saw palmetto berry, can produce results similar to Proscar. In my experience, this herb does seem to relieve symptoms associated with a large prostate in some patients. While I know of no evidence that it actually decreases the size of the prostate, I believe saw palmetto to be safe and worth a try. You can buy it in most drug stores without a prescription.

Surgical options
OPEN SURGERY AND TRANSURETHRAL RESECTION OF THE PROSTATE (TURP)

In the event that symptoms are progressive despite the use of medication, or in cases wherein the prostate is massively enlarged, surgical removal of the prostate gland may be necessary. Concern about potential sexual impotence following prostate surgery has struck fear into the hearts of many men. While these concerns are founded in reality, they are often exaggerated. Improved surgical techniques have significantly reduced the frequency of this complication. Depending on the size of the gland and the type of surgery required, the incidence of this unhappy result varies from less than five percent to less than 20 percent.

Open surgery has been the gold standard for most cases of advanced enlargement. In some cases, however, the gland can be removed with the use of small scopes *(laparoscopic prostatectomy)* inserted into the lower abdomen—and more recently with robotic surgical techniques. These procedures also appear to greatly diminish post-operative discomfort and complications.

When the gland is *not* massively enlarged, obstructing prostatic tissue can often be removed with the use of a small scope through the urethra. This lesser form of surgery is known as a *transurethral resection of the prostate* (TURP). The majority of patients who require surgery can be effectively treated with a TURP. Over the years, TURP has become one of the most commonly performed urological surgeries, and it gets high marks for good results.

DESTRUCTION OF EXCESS PROSTATE TISSUE

Given the successful track record of removing obstructing prostatic tissue through the urethra with a TURP, the advent of a number of new transurethral techniques should come as no surprise. In an effort to avoid the need for surgery, these techniques focus on the destruction rather than the removal of excessive prostatic tissue. Recently, *transurethral electrovaporization* of the prostate (TEVP) has grown in popularity. This procedure vaporizes the obstructing prostatic tissue with an electric current. While the procedure does require hospitalization and spinal or general anesthesia, it appears to result in fewer complications and shorter hospital stays than a TURP.

Similarly destructive procedures (using a variety of different modalities) are currently growing in popularity, because they can be done on an outpatient basis with local anesthesia. Some examples are *high-intensity ultrasound, transurethral microwave,* and *transurethral needle ablation.* One of the "newest kids" on the block is *water-induced thermotherapy* (WIT), which is also performed on an outpatient basis with local anesthesia. In selected cases, this has shown very promising results with minimal discomfort and no reports of sexual dysfunction.

Each one of these procedures has a cadre of enthusiastic physician advocates. For this reason, it's very important to understand that (1) a urinary catheter is required for a variable number of days after all of these techniques, and (2) one shoe does not fit all feet. If you need this kind of relief, be sure you have an experienced urological surgeon to help you decide which procedure is best for your particular case.

ERECTILE DYSFUNCTION

Erectile dysfunction (also referred to as ED) is an inability to achieve an erection or maintain an erection of sufficient quality to have sexual intercourse. There are a number of things that can cause this problem. Basically, however, they fall into two categories: psychological or physical—and sometimes both. To better understand ED, it's probably a good idea to briefly go over the anatomy of the penis and the normal mechanism of erection.

An erection occurs when the penis becomes engorged with blood. The engorgement and trapping of blood in the penis is what causes the penis to enlarge, get longer, and become more rigid. But this momentous event involves a series of highly complex reactions.

This illustration depicts both a cross-section and a longitudinal section of the penis. As you can see, the main bulk of the penis is made up of two spongelike structures known as the *corpus cavernosum* and the *corpus spongiosum*—the former being the larger of the two. These spongelike structures receive the blood supplied by the arteries of the penis. The veins of the penis drain the blood out of these sponges. The spaces in this spongelike tissue (called *sinusoids*) fill up with blood during an erection. As these spaces or sinusoids are expanding with blood, they compress the veins— the exit route of the blood from these sinusoids. With the exit channels closed, the blood is trapped in the sinusoids— expanding the penis and making it turgid.

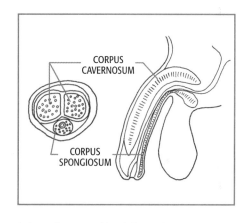

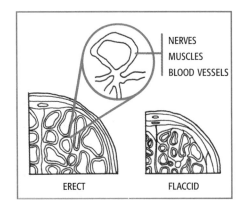

NERVES
MUSCLES
BLOOD VESSELS

ERECT   FLACCID

In between and around the sinusoids, there are tiny nerves and muscle fibers. When the penis is in its normal resting state, these little muscle fibers are contracted. When these tiny muscle fibers relax, the sinusoids become more elastic and are able to receive more blood. Bloodflow to the penis is increased by emotional, visual, or tactile stimulation. Messages transmitted by hormones and nerves signal the increase in bloodflow and tell the muscles in the penis to relax. This allows blood to fill and expand the sinusoids. As the sinusoids expand and enlarge, the veins—the channels that drain the sinusoids—are compressed. This traps the blood in the spongelike structures of the penis and causes an erection.

Now there's another important aspect of this process that I didn't mention—*neurotransmitters*.

Perhaps you remember our previous discussion about brain function. We talked about neurotransmitters such as serotonin, norepinephrine, and others. These chemicals are released by nerve endings that assist in transmitting messages from one nerve to another, or from a nerve to a muscle—telling it what to do. Probably, the most important neurotransmitter in the mechanism of erection is nitric oxide. The release of this substance triggers a series of events that causes the muscle in the spongelike structures to relax. And, as just explained, the relaxation of these muscles allows the sinusoids to open up and fill with more blood.

After an ejaculation or fatigue, the neurotransmitters are turned off, and those muscles in the spongelike structures contract into their normal resting state. This opens the venous channels, allowing the blood to be drained from the penis and the erection to fade. The penis returns to its inactive state.

THE CAUSES OF ERECTILE DYSFUNCTION IN OLDER MEN

While there are many causes for ED, for the purpose of our discussion let's focus our attention on those that are most relevant to the aging process: With advancing age, (1) the penis is less sensitive to touch and other forms of stimulation, (2) it takes a longer period of sexual stimulation to produce an erection, (3) erections are less firm and don't last as long, and (4) more recovery time is needed between erections.

Psychological versus physical problems

Sometimes the inability to get an erection is purely physical. In other cases it's caused by psychological problems such as the anxiety or depression that so often afflicts those of us with a chronic disease such as coronary artery disease or heart failure. Sometimes it's the result of the *fear of failure* factor previously discussed. Often, it's a combination of both—the physical as well as the psychological. When the cause is psychological, psychotherapy and treatment by sex therapists can be helpful.

Since an erection is the result of the penis becoming engorged with blood, it's clear that anything that limits bloodflow to the penis or decreases its ability to fill up presents a problem. The possible contributing factors are multiple. For example, arteriosclerosis associated with the aging process can interfere with bloodflow to the penis. Diabetes and cigarette smoking—because they advance arteriosclerosis—can make this worse. Scientists also suspect that, as we age, the muscle fibers in the spongy tissue of the penis increase in tone. This could make it more difficult for the spaces (sinusoids) in this spongy tissue to receive blood. Waning testosterone production, diminished sensitivity of the nerves of the penis, and a decrease in neurotransmitters also develop with aging.

And if *that's* not enough, we have to understand that many people are subject to a number of chronic diseases that may adversely affect erection. What's more, a number of the medications used to treat these conditions may also have an adverse effect on erection.

THE TREATMENT OF ERECTILE DYSFUNCTION

If you have ED, what can you do about it? The first thing you should do is see your doctor. He or she may make simple changes in your medication that can make all the difference in the world. In other instances, your doctor might recommend certain tests to identify the cause or causes of your ED. Having said that, let's discuss some of the treatments that have been used over the years.

Surgery

In the early 1970s, penile prostheses were in favor. This involved the surgical insertion, into the penis, of a device that kept the penis firm for the purpose of performing intercourse. Improvement in these devices enabled the penis to be pumped up or decompressed as desired. Among the disadvantages of this procedure were infection, malfunctioning of the prosthesis, and the very fact that a surgical implantation was required. Still, in the absence of a better solution, many men and their spouses opted to have the operation and a good number of them are still enjoying the results.

In the next decade, surgical procedures to improve the blood-flow to the penis became popular. Patients were studied to determine if there was a significant obstruction to the main artery to the penis. If there was, the obstruction was surgically remedied. This worked for some patients, but not for others. Why? Because, as already explained, the cause of ED in our aging member is usually due to several factors. Moreover, surgical improvement of circulation in the main artery did not necessarily improve bloodflow through the smaller branches.

Prostaglandins

Prostaglandins, often called nature's protective substances, are made naturally at several different locations in our body. For quite some time we've known that they play an important role in the process of erection. But to use them to treat ED, they must be administered either by a small needle injection directly into the side of the penis or by putting the medication into the urethra of the penis. This form of treatment can be highly successful when patients are carefully instructed in the self-administration of these agents. There are, however, some important drawbacks. Just to mention a few of them: the inconvenience and discomfort of administration, urethral pain, and *priapism* (a painful and persistent erection). Priapism can have serious consequences and, in some cases, may require emergency treatment. Fortunately, it is an uncommon side effect.

Testosterone

While it is sometimes useful when a patient's ED is associated with a marked deficiency in testosterone, treating with this hormone can have both long-term and short-term side effects. Testosterone injections have great activity during the first week after injection but decrease thereafter. This can result in a roller-coaster effect characterized by jubilance, excitement—and even aggressiveness—followed by periods of fatigue, lassitude, and sometimes severe depression.

Oral testosterone treatment (in pill form) has been a problem because the only kind thus far available in this country is *methyltestosterone*. This particular form of testosterone has been associated with the development of severe liver disease. However, more recently developed preparations of testosterone *undecanoate* are demonstrating good results with fewer hazards. The jury is still out on these and a number of other new preparations that are in the pipeline.

More recently developed testosterone skin patches have a much smoother effect than injection therapy. These patches can raise testosterone levels to normal in more than 90 percent of men.

Sometimes they cause annoying skin irritations, but the even newer gel-type preparations appear to have substantially solved this problem. An added benefit: These gel preparations also seem to have a very positive side effect on bone mineral density.

My major concern with testosterone replacement therapy has to do with the long-term effects as they relate to the prostate gland and the cardiovascular system. Testosterone may increase the growth of the prostate gland—a problem that should concern some of us older guys. As we've discussed, enlargement of the prostate gland can obstruct the neck of the urinary bladder—and in severe cases this may require remedial surgery.

The effect testosterone can have on prostate cancer is even more important. Why? Because it might make the cancer grow faster. Certainly, anyone with this form of cancer must avoid testosterone. *And suppose that some of us don't yet know that we have prostate cancer.* Suppose we're walking around with a small, undiagnosed prostate cancer that doesn't show up on blood tests and might otherwise be so slow-growing that it doesn't threaten our lives. Should we nourish and encourage the growth of this cancer with testosterone? I think not. *Caution must be exercised in using this stuff.* It's really important to have regular examinations of the prostate gland—both in the form of rectal exams and blood tests.

Testosterone can also raise serum lipids and in so doing promote the development of atherosclerosis and coronary artery disease. So if you're going to take testosterone, you should have your serum lipid levels checked at regular intervals.

Medications

A host of medications—including yohimbine, phentolamine, apomorphine, papaverine, trazodone—have been recommended for the treatment of ED. All of them have been used with some small degree of success, but most with some undesirable side effects. That said, none of these medications has had the impact and success of *sildenafil*—otherwise known as *Viagra*, which has proven to be very effective. Through a complex series of reactions, Viagra causes an increase in the concentration of nitric oxide in the penis. This relaxes the smooth muscles in the spongy tissue of the penis and allows the sinusoids to accept more blood and become more turgid. So there you have it: *correction of erection without injection;* it's a pill.

Viagra takes about an hour to start working—but after you take it, the medicine is usually effective for a period of four to five hours. It's sort of like going to an amusement park—a one-hour wait for a three-minute ride. I'm sure that faster-acting versions of similar drugs are being developed—perhaps in the form of a sublingual version or a nasal spray.

Longer-acting drugs of a similar nature (Cialis and Levitra) are also available. With the use of these agents, gentle sexual stimulation will most often produce a good erection. The usually mild side effects include nasal congestion, heartburn, headache, and flushing. For the most part, these are infrequent and transient. Even less frequently, visual disturbances and priapism (an erection lasting more than four hours) occur, requiring medical attention. Certain heart medications and blood pressure medicines do represent an important contraindication to this kind of therapy, and rare cardiac problems have been reported. For these reasons, it's important for your doctor to determine if this treatment is right for you. *Please don't get this stuff from the Internet or black market sources.* Be smart and check with your physician.

HORMONE REPLACEMENT THERAPY AND SEXUALITY IN WOMEN

As previously discussed, estrogen replacement therapy via pills or patches has many advantages in regard to sexuality—but there are also some very serious disadvantages. Surely, estrogen appears to improve vaginal lubrication, libido, and skin texture, and helps to combat insomnia in postmenopausal women. Some women find estrogen's ability to alleviate hot flashes and night sweats and to help prevent osteoporosis even more important. On the flip side, recent studies of women taking estrogen and progesterone have yielded disturbing results. An increase in the frequency of breast cancer, uterine cancer, ovarian cancer, strokes, and heart attacks has been suggested. Whether or not a woman should take estrogen is an individual decision that should not be taken lightly. *The pros and cons should be carefully discussed with your doctor.* Soy products and other plant estrogens as well as some herbs such as black cohosh may provide some of the benefits of estrogen replacement therapy without its attendant risks.

LOOKING BACK, LOOKING FORWARD

CHAPTER 17 REVIEW ···

- Men who deal with BPH (benign prostatic hyperplasia) can alleviate symptoms with medications or surgery.

- Treatments for both the psychological and physical causes of ED (erectile dysfunction) begin with a doctor's evaluation.

- Testosterone replacement therapy may help some with ED, but potentially serious long-term effects related to the prostate gland and the cardiovascular system are a concern.

- While hormone replacement therapy (HRT) can have some physical, mental, and sexual benefits, recent studies have shown disturbing side effects.

CHAPTER 18 PREVIEW ···

- How important are screening tests and vaccinations as we grow older? Can regular self-examinations really make a difference?

- What can be done about age-related hearing and vision problems? Are medications effective for these conditions, or is surgery always required?

- What screening tests can best protect us from colon cancer?

THE FOUNTAIN OF AGE

Age is not "lost youth" but a new stage of opportunity and strength.
—Betty Friedan

There is a fountain of youth: It is your mind, your
talents, the creativity you bring to your life and the
lives of the people you love. When you learn to
tap this source, you will truly have defeated age.
—Sophia Loren

The Spanish explorer Ponce de León didn't have much luck when he tried to find the fabled "Fountain of Youth" some 500 years ago. While searching deep in the jungles of Florida, his heart was fatally pierced by an arrow launched from a hostile native's bow. He was only 47 years old. The conclusion: We will do better by searching for the "Fountain of Age."

So, what does it really mean to "age gracefully"? To some, it means passively and pleasantly accepting the disabilities of advancing age. *But don't you believe it.* As Albert Einstein said, "Life is like riding a bicycle. To keep your balance, you should keep moving." The preceding chapters have made that point, haven't they? The truth is that it's crucial to be active rather than passive. Only in this way can we *compress morbidity*—the true and realistic definition of aging gracefully. That means staying healthy and independent for as long as possible—so you can continue to enjoy all of the magnificent wonders of life.

To this end, no discussion or series of discussions on the subject of aging and fitness would be complete without addressing some of the medical aspects of maintaining good health. To do your part, you must be aware of what the doctor must check out, and what you should check yourself. You must also make it your business to know what screening tests you should have performed and what vaccinations you need to maintain good health.

AN OUNCE OF PREVENTION

It's much easier to prevent some diseases than to cure them. Others, as I'm sure you can appreciate, can be most effectively cured when the problem is identified in its early stages. The two most important ways to achieve early detection are (1) awareness and self-examination, and (2) periodic health screening examinations. What's the best schedule for screening exams? It's the one arrived at by you and your doctor. Both of you should thoroughly discuss all the issues relating to your health status, your age, and the presence or absence of any diseases in your family that could affect your future. In addition to hereditary diseases, these include hereditary *tendencies* to develop problems such as heart disease, diabetes, colorectal cancer, breast cancer, and many others.

SELF-EXAMINATION OF THE GENITALS

Let's discuss self-examination and awareness as the first order of business. Women should examine their genital area, checking for lumps, sores, warts, or any abnormal vaginal discharge. All of these are warning signs that signal the need for medical consultation and advice.

Men should take note also. By looking and feeling, cancer of the penis can be easily diagnosed in its early stages. The same is true of testicular tumors. These tumors are not as common in older men as they are in younger men—and not nearly as common as breast cancer in women. But they *do* occur, and they can be diagnosed at an early stage by self-exam. So check your penis and carefully examine each testicle. If you feel any lumps or notice any increase in size, see your doctor.

SELF-EXAMINATION OF THE BREASTS

Now ladies—please, please, and please again, *you must examine your own breasts.* Don't rely on mammograms and doctor visits as the only source of detecting a lump. I can't tell you how many times I've seen patients with lumps in their breasts that proved to be cancer—cancer that didn't show up on mammography. *Mammograms are not foolproof, believe me.* I know that many women play the ostrich until they go to the doctor. But you can't do that. You can't be the ostrich, because the stakes are too high and the results of early detection and treatment of breast cancer are too good. You can't allow a preventable catastrophe to develop because of your fear of finding something—something that can be cured.

When you visit the doctor, make sure he or she does a breast examination as opposed to just ordering a mammogram. Again, mammography is a very good test—but it's not foolproof. While

I urge you to ask your doctor to show you the preferred way to self-examine your breasts, here are a few tips. First, look at your breasts, and then look at them again in a mirror. Use a good mirror in a well-lit room and study your breasts from different angles. Stand in front of the mirror with your hands behind your head, again with your hands on your hips, and then one more time while bending slightly forward so that your breasts hang freely. See if you can detect any lumps, any retraction or inversion of the nipple, any kind of skin changes, or any difference in the motion between the two breasts. Don't be alarmed if one breast appears slightly larger than the other; that's not uncommon.

Next, feel your breasts. Get used to the way your breasts feel so that if changes develop, you can detect them. It's a good idea to feel your breasts in two positions: lying down and standing up (perhaps while showering). Don't use the end of your fingertips; use the flat ends of your fingers. The skin on the undersurface at the end of your fingers is much more sensitive to touch than the skin on the very tips of your fingers. While doing the exam, it can be helpful to use a little lubricant or moisturizing lotion or soap and water on your hands. This decreases the friction of your fingers against the skin and increases your ability to detect changes.

Divide the breast into four quadrants: the upper-outer, the upper-inner, the lower-outer, and the lower-inner quadrants. Examine each quadrant of each breast thoroughly by systematically using gentle pressure in small circular, searching movements. Examine your left breast with your right hand while your left hand is raised behind your head. Then, reverse the position of your hands to examine your right breast. After you've done that, be sure to check deep in each armpit or *axilla* for lumps. To do this, put your fingers in your axilla (your armpit) and then lower your arm. This reduces the tension of the muscles that make up the armpit. With your fingers now placed deep in your armpit, repeat the same gentle circular examination.

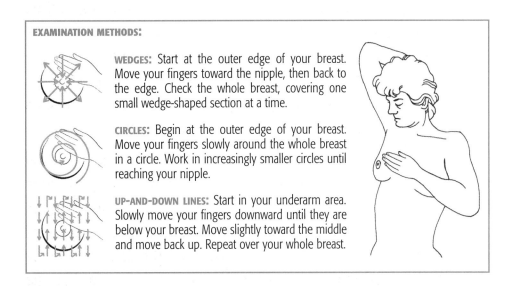

EXAMINATION METHODS:

WEDGES: Start at the outer edge of your breast. Move your fingers toward the nipple, then back to the edge. Check the whole breast, covering one small wedge-shaped section at a time.

CIRCLES: Begin at the outer edge of your breast. Move your fingers slowly around the whole breast in a circle. Work in increasingly smaller circles until reaching your nipple.

UP-AND-DOWN LINES: Start in your underarm area. Slowly move your fingers downward until they are below your breast. Move slightly toward the middle and move back up. Repeat over your whole breast.

Next, carefully check each nipple for any skin changes. Then gently squeeze each nipple between your thumb and index finger and check for a discharge.

A cloudy discharge caused by squeezing the nipple is usually normal—but if it's bloody or brown, you should check with your doctor. Suppose you feel something? First of all, remember that most lumps are not cancers. Often they're cysts or benign tumors, *but they may be cancers.* So if you find a lump or anything that puzzles you, get a professional opinion. Another thing—if you find a lump that feels tender, don't disregard it. It's true that cancers are not usually tender, but on some occasions, they are.

"Clumps of lumps" can be the norm for many women. In fact, most women have some lumpiness or areas of thickness in their breasts. If it's the same on both sides, it's probably not significant. Check with your doctor if you notice any of the following: Your findings are not the same on each side, you feel something that's different from what you usually feel, or you feel an area that is harder than the rest of your breast.

For those of you who are menstruating, it's a good idea to do your examinations a few days *after* your menstrual period (when your breasts have returned to normal and are less engorged and swollen).

Men should also be doing a self-examination of their chests. Although breast cancer is unusual in men, it *does* happen—so it makes sense to check yourself out, using the same method described for the ladies.

MAMMOGRAMS, ULTRASOUND, AND MRI

Mammograms are special breast x-rays that can detect tumors that are too small to feel—but let me repeat that *they're not foolproof*. Mammography should not be viewed as a substitute for clinical exams by your physician or for the frequent self-examinations previously recommended. Mammograms should be an addition to them. Also, if you know you have a lump, please tell your doctor right away. In such cases, your mammogram might be coupled with an ultrasound and/or a magnetic resonance imaging (MRI) examination of the breasts and the suspicious area in question. Remember that mammograms are important—but they're not foolproof.

Many authorities recommend that women start yearly mammograms at age 50, but in my opinion, they are best started at age 40. On the other hand—if a close relative, such as your mother or sister, developed breast cancer in their thirties or forties, I think you should consider starting your mammograms and doctor examinations even earlier. Women who are at particular risk, such as those who have a family history of the disease or those who might already have had breast cancer, should usually have the additional screening that can be provided by an MRI. In some cases, genetic testing can also help to determine your level of risk. *Please, ladies, discuss this with your doctor.* And remember—while all examinations are less than perfect, early diagnosis coupled with prompt treatment is your best chance to be cured.

CERVICAL CANCER SCREENING AND PELVIC EXAMINATIONS

As all of you know, a pelvic examination is an internal vaginal examination by your doctor. In addition to visually inspecting your external genitalia, the doctor will do a bimanual examination with two fingers of one hand in the vagina and the other hand on the lower abdomen. In this way, he or she can search for abnormalities involving the uterus and ovaries. Next, the doctor will insert a speculum into the vagina to visually examine the vagina and the cervix of the uterus. At this time the doctor will perform a Pap smear test for cancer of the cervix. It's recommended that a Pap test be done every one to three years. The proper frequency of these examinations *for you* can best be determined in consultation with your doctor. An example: If you have significant risk factors, such as a history of genital warts or a family history of cervical cancer, it might be more appropriate for you to have the test annually. If, on the other hand, you don't have any risk factors—or if you've had a hysterectomy for reasons other than uterine or cervical cancer—you may not need annual exams. It should be noted that most cancers of the cervix are related to the human papillomavirus (HPV), the same virus that causes genital warts. Recently a vaccine has been developed that, if given in youth, will substantially decrease the frequency of cervical cancer.

PROSTATE CANCER SCREENING

Prostate cancer is one of the more common causes of death in older men. The good news is that it's usually curable when detected and treated in the early stages. In some cases, there appears to be a family predisposition to prostate cancer, and it also seems more common in men who eat a high-fat diet and men of African-American descent. The cancer usually develops after the age of 65, but it can occur earlier. In my opinion, initial screening should begin between the ages of 45 and 50. How is prostate cancer screened? By digital rectal examination and by means of a blood test known as the PSA (prostate specific antigen). This substance circulates in the blood in two forms; one is bound to a protein, and the other is free, or unbound. Sometimes equivocal results in the total PSA can be clarified by determining the ratio of free PSA to bound PSA. Free PSA should be 20 percent or more of the total PSA. Because no test is foolproof, have both the digital rectal exam *and* the blood test done every year. If an abnormality is detected, your doctor may want to do a biopsy. This is done through the rectum with the use of an ultrasound device that permits the targeting of several punch biopsies. (But don't get frightened, boys. Although this procedure may be a little uncomfortable, it's not really painful.)

It's useful to note that the disease appears to be less dangerous in older men. In this case it often grows more slowly and may not significantly affect longevity. Prostate cancer is more serious when contracted between the late 40s and the early 70s, and it appears to gradually decrease in severity with advancing age. That's why many authorities question the value of routine screening of older gentlemen.

THE PARTNERSHIP WITH YOUR DOCTOR

What additional health checkups and vaccinations should you expect from your doctor? This decision depends on your age, your risk factors, and the state of your health. Let's focus on some of the issues for which careful monitoring would be of most benefit to mature and older adults.

BLOOD PRESSURE

High blood pressure, also known as *hypertension*, is a real killer. It's associated with a high incidence of strokes, heart attacks, and congestive heart failure. Contrary to popular belief, it's not usually symptomatic. Most people with high blood pressure don't even know they have it. They have no headaches, dizziness, or any symptoms at all. Instead, this disease quietly progresses, like a thief in the night, to produce its ill effects.

That's why you must have your blood pressure checked. If it's elevated, you should discuss the treatment options with your doctor. Sometimes the treatment is quite simple, involving lifestyle modifications such as weight reduction, salt restriction, and exercise. At other times, medication is required. *The first and most important step is to know about it if you have it.* So get your blood pressure checked. If it's elevated, have it taken care of and keep a careful check on it.

The risk of developing high blood pressure is greater if there's a history of hypertension, strokes, or heart disease in your family or if you are of African-American descent. While all of us should have our blood pressure checked at least once a year, if you're at high risk or if you already know you have high blood pressure, the frequency of your pressure checks should be decided in consultation with your doctor. Relatively inexpensive and convenient home blood pressure machines are readily available to enable those of you in these situations to monitor your own blood pressure at frequent intervals. This information can be of great value to the decision-making process you share with your physician.

VISION EVALUATION

The older we get the less well we are able to see. While I'm not offering you a course in ophthalmology, I do want to discuss some of the more common difficulties we experience with our aging eyes.

Presbyopia

Needless to say, your sight is one of your most precious assets. Regardless of the cause, visual impairments can affect your balance and your ability to walk, negotiate stairs, and avoid falls. All of us realize that our visual acuity changes as we get older. For the most part, however, it can be corrected. As we age, the lens becomes less pliable and less able to change its shape to accommodate for near objects. This part of the aging process is given the fancy name of *presbyopia*. While this change in visual accommodation actually begins in our teens, we usually don't require corrective lenses until we're 40 years old or older. So if you're beginning to have difficulty reading fine print, *get your vision checked*. A good pair of spectacles can make a world of difference and save you a lot of grief.

Cataracts

Cataracts are opacities that "cloud" the clarity of the eye's lens like a spot on the lens of your eyeglasses. While many factors contribute to cataracts, they are usually the consequence of the degenerative changes that occur with aging. Cataracts cause a progressive and painless loss of vision. Frequent changes in eyeglass prescriptions can often maintain useful vision. When this fails, surgery can usually produce excellent results.

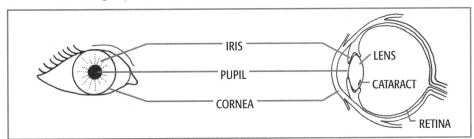

Glaucoma

Glaucoma is a condition characterized by an increase of pressure within the eyeball. It usually comes on gradually, but it may develop suddenly—and it can cause anything from slightly impaired vision to complete blindness. What symptoms sound an alert? Seeing a halo around electric lights, pain or pressure in an eye, headaches, and vague visual disturbances. Those at greatest risk are people older than age 35, those with a family history of glaucoma, and patients with diabetes. While there are different types of glaucoma and many causes for it, glaucoma is usually an easy diagnosis for your ophthalmologist to make. The good news is that the majority of cases can be adequately treated with medicine or surgery.

Macular degeneration

A more troublesome condition is age-related macular degeneration (AMD), which is the leading cause of serious visual impairment in the elderly. It produces a progressive loss of central vision, and while the onset is usually gradual, it might also be catastrophically sudden. A National Eye Institute study found that, by taking high-dose antioxidant vitamins (vitamins C and E, beta-carotene, zinc, and copper), those most at risk reduce the progression to advanced AMD by 25 percent and the risk of moderate vision loss by 19 percent. Researchers also found that people who engage in regular exercise were less likely to develop AMD. The bottom line? A healthy lifestyle, quitting smoking, and a diet rich in green leafy vegetables and fish is the way to go.

Although there is no adequate medical treatment for AMD, laser therapy can occasionally help cases that are identified early. Intensive research in gene therapy is under way to find a cure or a method of prevention. Hopefully, a breakthrough is not far away.

Diabetic retinopathy

As its name implies, a deterioration of the retina called *diabetic retinopathy* is a major cause of blindness in people with diabetes, and it's made worse by hypertension. Careful control of diabetes and blood pressure is *crucial* in retarding or preventing this problem. While the condition can't be reversed after it's established, when it's identified early, laser therapy can sometimes produce improvement.

• • •

I've only just touched on the myriad of problems that affect the eyes. *But I want to emphasize the importance of regular vision checkups and eye examinations.* If you haven't been checked in a while, schedule them with your doctor. Diabetic patients, in particular, should have their eyes checked at least once a year by an ophthalmologist. These examinations should include a visual acuity evaluation, eye pressure measurements, and a thorough examination of the retina. What should you do if you develop visual difficulty or eye pain or eye pressure between your scheduled examinations? Seek medical advice as soon as possible.

The correction of visual problems by means of laser therapy (and more recently radiotherapy) has received wide public attention. Surgical techniques using lasers have allowed many folks to give up their glasses. The procedure is quick, relatively painless, and reportedly has a low incidence of complications. While this form of treatment has been effective for many conditions, it has not yet proven to counteract presbyopia. Further improvement in equipment and refinement in techniques are anticipated. Still investigational, radiotherapy has recently been used to change the convexity of the cornea—enabling some people to read without glasses. Both laser treatment and radiotherapy are likely to be particularly appealing to those who dislike wearing glasses. Their long-term benefits have not yet been completely evaluated, however, and we look forward to the results of future studies with great hope.

HEARING EVALUATION

Many diseases that cause hearing loss can be successfully treated—a good reason to get your hearing checked.

Presbycusis

Presbycusis, the form of hearing loss most often associated with aging, causes progressive hearing loss in older people as some of the structures of the inner ear stiffen and deteriorate. Some of us may become severely impaired by the time we're 60, while others seem relatively unscathed even into their 90s. The degree of impairment is highly variable.

Who is at greatest risk for presbycusis? People who've had prolonged exposure to loud noise in the workplace or who've habitually listened to loud music seem more likely to develop it earlier and possibly even more severely. This may be one of the reasons it's more common in men. The more interesting thing about this condition, however, is the victim's failure to recognize it in its early stages. Perhaps that's because it progresses so slowly, or simply because of denial—you know, *"I'm not hard of hearing—not me."* Commonly, relatives or friends notice the situation first. But it's firmly denied when they mention it to the afflicted.

For the many of us who suffer from hearing loss, it's important to accept that it's a common consequence of aging—nothing to be ashamed of. In fact, *not* admitting it negatively affects your life in many ways. There are parts of conversations you're losing or not understanding—either because you don't hear them correctly, or because you don't hear enough of what was being said to understand it. The result? You might misinterpret parts of a conversation and then make a comment that's totally out of context. If your companions don't know about your problem, they may well think you're less intelligent than you really are. Even worse, they may decide that you're losing it a little, or conclude that you've turned into a doddering old fool who can be easily deceived.

More importantly, the input to your knowledge base is at least partially cut off. If you don't hear what you're intended to hear, you won't know some of the things you should know. You'll be less knowledgeable than you should be and less valuable than you could be. But you're not an old fool; you're not demented; *you just can't hear.*

Equally important is the isolation that hearing loss can impose on you. As the loss escalates, people often begin to "drop out."

Social activities such as weekly card games or dining with friends go from pleasurable to difficult—or even embarrassing. So you stop going. You misunderstand a comment made by a friend, and a friendship ends. Friends and family get tired of hearing you say, "Huh?" and begin to react with annoyance, frustration, or even anger. The result? You can eventually find yourself isolated and alone—for no good reason!

So what should you do if your loved ones say they think you're having a hearing problem? *First, you should thank them.* Then, for God's sake, get your ears and hearing checked. You might be a good candidate for a hearing aid. If you are, go get one. Many of these newer devices are small, comfortable, more effective, and more easily concealed than the older versions. And if you need a larger version, so what! Don't let a false sense of ego stand in the way of your awareness, compromise your ability to learn and internalize new information, or lead you to a life of lonely isolation. Even more promising is the development of a device that can be surgically implanted. This is still in the developmental stage, but it holds great promise for the future.

Have you heard the story of the 95-year-old man with big thick eyeglasses and large hearing aids in each ear who was wandering the streets of New York? As he got more and more confused, the old fellow walked into St. Patrick's Cathedral and sat down in a confessional booth. The priest on the other side of the partition said, "Tell me, my son—how can I help you?" Hearing not a word, the old man didn't reply. The priest repeated this greeting several times, but after getting no answer he became frustrated and started banging on the partition—to which the old man responded, "Listen, buddy. You can stop the knocking and the banging, because there's no paper in this booth either."

Tinnitus

Tinnitus, a very common problem, can wear many different costumes. Sometimes it's a ringing, a hissing, a roaring, or some other kind of sound—like a buzzing. The sound can be constant or intermittent, and most people find it particularly annoying at night when they're lying in bed—probably because the sounds of the day don't block it out. The actual cause of tinnitus is obscure. Most of the time it's benign, or unrelated to a serious condition. What we do know is that it can be associated with almost any disorder of the ear, nose, or throat or even disturbances in other systems—such as the cardiovascular system. Immoderate tobacco use and even some medications—aspirin, for one—have been blamed. Tinnitus is also commonly associated with some degree of hearing loss. So people with tinnitus should have their hearing checked along with a thorough examination of their ears, nose, and throat. As I said before, there is no identifiable cause for the common, benign type of tinnitus, and there are no serious diseases associated with it. That's the good news. The bad news is that there is no known cure. Rest, avoidance of stress, cessation of smoking, medication changes, and the like have all met with varying degrees of success. Sometimes, sound-blocking devices can be of benefit.

COLORECTAL CANCER SCREENING

Colon cancer is one of the more common killers in our society. Most of these lethal cancers begin as benign polyps (noncancerous growths) that can be removed through a colonoscope. When cancer does develop, the cure rates from surgery are very good—*providing a diagnosis is made early.*

Early diagnosis and cure can be achieved through screening tests. These screening tests involve checking the stool for the presence of blood, examining the colon with x-ray studies, and examining the colon by direct visualization with the use of flexible instruments.

Fecal occult blood test

Most experts recommend that, after the age of 50, your stool should be tested once a year for the presence of blood. This fecal occult blood test is called an FOBT for short. Getting a positive test result doesn't mean you have cancer or a polyp, but having a negative result doesn't necessarily mean that you *don't* have one. Nonetheless, the FOBT appears to be a useful screening test to identify patients at high risk and is used to encourage further evaluation when necessary.

Flexible sigmoidoscopy and colonoscopy

Most experts also recommend a flexible sigmoidoscopy after the age of 50. But they disagree on how frequently this test should be performed after that. Opinions range from every three to every ten years. These differences in opinion have yet to be resolved— but they don't apply to people in a high-risk category. Individuals with a family history of colon cancer or colon polyps in a first- or second-degree relative and those who have colon disorders, such as ulcerative colitis, are examples of patients at higher risk.

Most would agree that individuals who are at high risk for developing colon cancer should have a complete colonoscopy, not just a flexible sigmoidoscopy. This procedure should be done about every three to five years.

A word of caution: If your father, mother, brother, or sister developed colon cancer, you should probably start your checkups 10 years before the diagnosis was made in that relative. The bottom line? *The age at which you start your checkups and the type of evaluation that should be performed is often related to your individual risk factors.*

What's the difference between the two tests? A flexible sigmoidoscopy is a shorter examination that checks your rectum and your sigmoid colon—the lower part of your colon. The instrument is inserted into the rectum and advanced into the sigmoid colon under video visualization. The length of the instrument is usually 65 centimeters, so it can be used to examine about 25 inches of the lower colon and the rectum. Most people say that the examination is a little uncomfortable, but not usually painful. In selected instances, your doctor might recommend a barium enema (a lower GI x-ray study) to examine the rest of your colon.

A colonoscopy is done with a longer instrument because its purpose is to examine the entire colon. This examination requires a more extensive preparation, including laxatives and a day or two of dietary restrictions. It's usually done with the use of sedation and pain medication.

Because of the excellent sedation that's normally used for colonoscopy, the procedure is rarely painful. After it's over, most people don't even remember it. The most difficult part of the whole procedure is the preparation—and that's not all that bad.

Virtual colonoscopy

A promising development on the horizon is called *virtual colonoscopy*. This test can be performed painlessly and quickly, as it examines the colon with a special CT x-ray. While the technique is still undergoing study and improvement, it seems likely to become a cost-effective, less uncomfortable, and much more convenient way to screen most people for colon tumors in the not too distant future.

CHOLESTEROL AND BLOOD SUGAR DETERMINATIONS

We've already talked about the importance of your blood cholesterol and the desirable ranges for total cholesterol and for HDL and LDL. But when should you start to have these checked? Most authorities feel that men should start annual cholesterol screening at age 35 and continue it through age 65 or longer. Women should do the same, starting at age 45.

These general mandates are not specific to all individuals, however. You may have one of many risk factors that indicate the need to have your cholesterol checked earlier and more frequently. To mention a few: If you have a family history of early heart attack, if you have a history of tobacco use, if your cholesterol is elevated, if you have diabetes, or if you have high blood pressure, you're in a higher-risk group.

These risk factors are important and need to be clearly identified and discussed with your physician. The same is true for your blood sugar. Anyone can get diabetes—and there's a much greater likelihood of this happening to you if you have a family history of diabetes, if you're overweight, or if you eat a lot of sugar. So get your blood sugar checked.

C-REACTIVE PROTEIN (CRP)

Now let me call your attention to a related issue. Many authorities believe that inflammation plays an important role in the development of heart attacks. To check this belief, they measured markers in the blood for inflammation and found them to be elevated in many people who went on to have a heart attack—even in the presence of normal levels of bad cholesterol.

These markers, in the absence of other causes for inflammation such as infection or recent trauma, appear to be quite accurate predictors of cardiac risk. One of the best tests of these markers is the determination of the CRP, otherwise known as *C-reactive protein*. This blood test is readily available and easily performed. You might ask your doctor about adding it to your usual cardiac risk assessment.

FLU AND PNEUMONIA VACCINATIONS

So far so good. Now let's talk a little about vaccination as it applies to us older folks.

Older adults—and particularly those with chronic pulmonary or cardiac conditions—are very susceptible to the complications of the flu and to pneumonia. The Centers for Disease Control (CDC) has done a wonderful job of predicting the particular strain of flu viruses that are most likely to hit us each year. They've missed from time to time—but no one is perfect, and they're getting better and better at it. Based on these predictions, a new flu vaccine that usually protects against three different viruses is produced each year. That's why flu shots are sometimes in short supply. It takes several weeks to develop immunity after receiving the vaccine, but the immunity lasts for about six months. I highly recommend that older adults take this shot every year unless their doctor suggests otherwise. He or she may recommend against it because you have a history of adverse reactions or an allergy.

Pneumonia vaccinations are available for a particular kind of this disease known as *pneumococcal pneumonia*—not for all kinds of pneumonia. Among older adults, pneumococcal pneumonia is responsible for numerous deaths each year. At one time this vaccination was recommended as a once-in-a-lifetime shot. Now, however, most authorities suggest that it be repeated every three to five years. I urge you to take this shot and save yourself the misery of a very serious illness.

CONTROVERSY OVER PREVENTATIVE HEALTH-SCREENING IN THE ELDERLY

Did you know there's a great deal of controversy as to the efficacy of cholesterol and cancer screening in older age groups? It's true. Preventative health-screening tests and periodic physical examinations, in general, have come under scrutiny—particularly in the elderly. In the minds of some authorities, the costs and the disparity between supply and demand have indicated the need for rationing medical services—even some vaccines. They point to the minimal statistical benefit that can be expected from some of these screening tests as a reason to restrict them to younger people. For example: Statistics demonstrate that the average 75-year-old will most likely live another 12 years, so giving up Pap smears would result in an average loss of only three days of life expectancy. Also, giving up mammograms and fecal occult blood tests at this age would be at a statistical cost of only nine days of longevity. Even abandoning the routine use of mammograms at the very early age of 50 seems to come at a cost of only 43 days of longevity—a difference of just six weeks.

Do these statistically derived findings justify doing these screening tests? Maybe not—not on the face of it. But that's not what health-screening tests are about. These are averages—and as such, they're not applicable to individuals.

I say this: *If you're going to do something about a disease when you diagnose it, you should do screening tests for it.* A good example is a patient of mine named Marjorie. Although she didn't know her family history at the time of her own ordeal, we later found that her mother had died of colon cancer at the age of 83. Even later, it was determined that her aunt also succumbed to colon cancer at the age of 85. Marjorie was luckier—because we found her colon cancer at the age of 82 by doing a routine screening test for blood in the stool. Her positive test result led to a colonoscopy which identified the cancer and led to a successful surgical cure. It's now 14 years later. Marjorie is 96 years old and still living independently in her own apartment— all because of a screening test for blood in the stool.

Health screening tests are performed to identify those individuals who can benefit from early diagnosis and treatment. Clearly, it makes no sense to screen for diseases that are unlikely to occur in the older age groups—such as chlamydia and gonorrhea. And it also makes no sense to screen for a disease for which the treatment would pose a greater threat to the individual than the disease itself.

The question we must always ask is whether or not the algebraic sum of the benefits outweighs the hazards of diagnosis and treatment for a given condition in a given individual. If the answer to that question is yes, and there is a simple screening test for that disease, then the test should be made available to that individual. To do otherwise—*to apply statistical averages to an individual based on age—imbeds age discrimination into health care policy.*

If a 75-year-old individual has a projected life expectancy of 12 or 20 years instead of two years, then surely he or she should have selected screening tests. On the other hand, if a less healthy 55-year-old individual has a life expectancy of only three or five years, perhaps certain screening tests don't make sense.

Now add to this discussion the likelihood of further increases in functional longevity. Might we not find a cure for Alzheimer's disease during the next 10 years? Can we not decrease the frequency of falls—perhaps by 50 percent— through strength and balance training programs? Might we not discover newer and better anti-aging treatments through investigating the human genome and stem cell research? *These are real possibilities—not pie in the sky.* When one realizes how dramatically these changes could alter the equation, the rigorous prevention of disease and screening tests in older adults enters a new and positive dimension.

Statistics can sometimes be likened to a drunk person leaning on a lamppost, i.e., *used more for support than enlightenment.* All of us must be cautiously aware of how a well-meaning scientific community's statistical efforts can be improperly construed—and thus create programs that discriminate against the aged.

Remember that each and every one of us can be Nifty after Fifty and "win in the second half." So don't be disheartened when you feel the pain of getting old or when others imply that you're too old. When things are not quite as good as they could be, dig down a little deeper. You can rewind your mind; you can rewind your strength; you can rewind your balance and your flexibility. Most importantly, you can rewind your vitality and love of life. *You can do it.*

I believe this poem, "The Great Rewind," sums it all up.

The Great Rewind

In ways, I am told,
I'm getting too old,
That my brain is too dim,
And my thoughts are too grim.

While I'm certain to die,
When my years have passed by,
I still pray that my Keeper,
Will stay the Grim Reaper.

But the Reaper's distraction,
Depends on my action,
And the choices I make,
To secure my stake.

So, I'll summon the gumption,
To control my consumption,
And make myself stronger,
To keep fit yet longer.

I'll gather the grit,
To sharpen and restore my wit,
And harvest the hustle,
To strengthen and rebuild my muscle.

Then when my strength does rewind
And as well, my mind,
I will clearly behold
That the rest can be gold.

NOTES

NOTES